Long-Term Care

Guest Editor

LINDA G. DUMAS, PhD, RN, ANP-BC

NURSING CLINICS
OF NORTH AMERICA

www.nursing.theclinics.com

Consulting Editor
SUZANNE S. PREVOST, RN, PhD, COI

June 2009 • Volume 44 • Number 2

SAUNDERS an imprint of ELSEVIER, Inc.

W.B. SAUNDERS COMPANY

A Division of Elsevier Inc.

1600 John F. Kennedy Blvd., Suite 1800 • Philadelphia, PA 19103-2899

http://www.theclinics.com

NURSING CLINICS OF NORTH AMERICA Volume 44, Number 2
June 2009 ISSN 0029-6465, ISBN-13: 978-1-4377-0509-6, ISBN-10: 1-4377-0509-X

Editor: Katie Hartner
Developmental Editor: Donald Mumford

Nursing Clinics of North America (ISSN 0029-6465) is published quarterly by Elsevier Inc., 360 Park Avenue South, New York, NY 10010-1710. Months of issue are March, June, September, and December. Business and Editorial Offices: 1600 John F. Kennedy Blvd., Suite 1800, Philadelphia, PA 19103-2899. Periodicals postage paid at New York, NY and additional mailing offices. Subscription price per year is, $133.00 (US individuals), $273.00 (US institutions), $228.00 (international individuals), $334.00 (international institutions), $184.00 (Canadian individuals), $334.00 (Canadian institutions), $70.00 (US students), and $115.00 (international students). To receive student/resident rate, orders must be accompanied by name of affiliated institution, date of term, and the signature of program/residency coordinator on institution letterhead. Orders will be billed at individual rate until proof of status is received. Foreign air speed delivery is included in all *Clinics* subscription prices. All prices are subject to change without notice. **POSTMASTER:** Send address changes to *Nursing Clinics*, Elsevier Periodicals Customer Service, 11830 Westline Industrial Drive, St. Louis, MO 63146. **Customer Service: 1-800-654-2452 (US). From outside the United States, call 1-314-453-7041. Fax: 1-314-453-5170. E-mail: JournalsCustomerService-usa@elsevier.com** (for print support) and **JournalsOnlineSupport-usa @elsevier.com** (for online support).

Nursing Clinics of North America is covered in *EMBASE/Excerpta Medica, MEDLINE/PubMed (Index Medicus), Social Sciences Citation Index, Current Contents, ASCA, Cumulative Index to Nursing, RNdex Top 100,* and Allied Health Literature and International Nursing Index (INI).

Printed and bound by CPI Group (UK) Ltd, Croydon, CR0 4YY

Transferred to Digital Print 2011

Contributors

CONSULTING EDITOR

SUZANNE S. PREVOST, RN, PhD, COI
Associate Dean, Practice and Community Engagement, University of Kentucky, Lexington, Kentucky

GUEST EDITOR

LINDA G. DUMAS, PhD, RN, ANP-BC
Associate Professor of Nursing, College of Nursing and Health Sciences, University of Massachusetts Boston, Boston, Massachusetts

AUTHORS

CAROLYN BLANKS, BA
Vice President, Labor & Workforce Development, Massachusetts Senior Care Association, Newton Lower Falls, Massachusetts

JACKIE CROSSEN-SILLS, PT, PhD
Director of Program Development, Norwell VNA and Hospice, Norwell, Massachusetts

MARY (MEG) E. DOHERTY, MSN, ANP-BC, MBA
Norwell Visiting Nurse and Hospice, Norwell, Massachusetts

LINDA G. DUMAS, PhD, RN, ANP-BC
Associate Professor of Nursing, College of Nursing and Health Sciences, University of Massachusetts Boston, Boston, Massachusetts

BETH LOOMIS, MDiv
Director of Pastoral Care, Mount Auburn Hospital, Cambridge, Massachusetts

BARBARA MESSINGER-RAPPORT, MD, PhD, CMD, FACP
Acting Head and Assistant Professor, Section of Geriatric Medicine, Cleveland Clinic Lerner College of Medicine, Case Western Reserve University, Cleveland, Ohio

VICTORIA PALMER-ERBS, PhD, RN
Associate Professor of Nursing, University of Massachusetts Boston, College of Nursing and Health Sciences, Boston, Massachusetts

FRANCES L. PORTNOY, RN, MA, MS, PhD
Professor Emerita, University of Massachusetts Boston, College of Nursing and Health Sciences, Boston, Massachusetts

MURALI RAMADURAI, MD, CMD
Diplomate, American Board of Internal Medicine; and Diplomate, American Board of Hospice and Palliative Medicine, Senior Health Care Associates, Inc., Newton, Massachusetts

SUSAN C. REINHARD, PhD, RN, FAAN
Senior Vice President and Director, AARP Public Policy Institute; and Chief Strategist, Center to Champion Nursing in America, Washington, DC

KAREN M. ROBINSON, DNS, PMHCNS-BC, FAAN
Professor, University of Louisville School of Nursing, Louisville, Kentucky

IRENE TOOMEY, RN, MBA
Director of Performance Improvement, Norwell VNA and Hospice, Norwell, Massachusetts

JOAN F. WRIGHT, BA
Community Development Coordinator/Hospice Volunteer Coordinator, Norwell Visiting Nurse Association and Hospice, Norwell, Massachusetts

HEATHER M. YOUNG, PhD, RN, FAAN
Associate Vice Chancellor for Nursing, Betty Irene Moore School of Nursing, UC Davis Health System, Sacramento, California

Contents

> Nurses play an essential role in long-term care (LTC). They can and should do more to create the kind of services and supports that people seek for themselves and for their families. To provide this crucial leadership, nurses must understand and advocate the array of services and programs that fall within the term "LTC," including, but not limited to, "nursing home care." We need to reframe how we think about LTC so that we can be part of changing it for ourselves, as professional providers and future consumers.

> This article is about nursing leadership, workforce diversity, and underrepresentation in nursing. It is about long-term care, specifically the nursing home, the nurses, and the certified nursing assistants. The nursing shortage, the shortage of nurse educators, and curricular changes in the colleges and universities are *not* the focus of this work. The questions asked here are, *who* will care for the residents in nursing homes, and how will they recruit the much-needed leadership at a time of unprecedented need?

> Health disparities exist in long-term care as well as in the community. Disparities in healthcare typically result from the interplay of insurance; healthcare access; health literacy and cultural disparities; and geographic distribution. Residence in the nursing home complicates the situation since it introduces facility differences, regulations, and payer issues. This article offers two vignettes of residents that illustrate management of chronic issues, and addressing end of life concerns.

Part II

Part III

Mary E. Doherty

Hospice care has ancient origins, but its modern history has included a re-
surgence since the 1960s. Coverage of hospice care by Medicare and
other insurers has helped it develop into an important part of today's health
care system. Nevertheless, substantial barriers to its ideal use remain. This
article discusses those barriers, with an emphasis on organizational and
policy considerations. Hospice providers have an opportunity to educate
physicians, patients, and families and thus help them to make full use of
hospice care's potential.

Jackie Crossen-Sills, Irene Toomey, and Mary E. Doherty

The national healthcare agenda to improve efficiencies, reduce costs, provide high quality evidence and performance based care while simultaneously meeting stricter legal and regulatory requirements, has forced
home care and hospice staff to change the way they work. These pressures require a reliance on new technologies to meet these goals. Through
the agency-wide introduction and implementation of a variety of technological systems; electronic medical record/ point of care devises, telehealth, telephony and e-learning the Norwell VNA and Hospice has been
able to improve efficiencies for employees allowing the focus of services
to remain solely on patients and patient care. The technology has enhanced the agency's performance standards, communication and ultimate outcomes.

Frances L. Portnoy

The challenges to long-term care come from many directions. In this article, the focus is on the changing nature of expectations and experiences of
aging in three generations of a middle class family. This personal account
details the way in which these generational expectations have changed,
and what the long-term care system provides. Continuing care communities provide a setting for the older generation, but changing economic circumstances raise questions about how society will provide adequate long-
term care for the next cohort of elders.

> During the next 50 years, demographic aging—including graying of the baby boomers, increased longevity, and lower fertility rates—will change the needs for long-term care in the United States. These trends will have a great impact on the federal budget related to spending for Social Security, Medicare, and Medicaid. Future years will see a more diverse population with increased aggressive treatment of chronic illness. Consumers of health care and their family caregivers will take more active steps to manage and coordinate their own care. Housing trends that produce more senior-friendly communities will encourage independent living rather than seniors' having to move into institutions; increased incentives for use of home- and community community-based care will allow people to stay longer in their own homes in the community. Technological advances, such as the use of robots who serve as companions and assistants around the house, will also decrease the need for institutional living.

THE CLINICS ARE NOW AVAILABLE ONLINE!

Access your subscription at:
www.theclinics.com

Preface

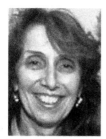

Linda G. Dumas, PhD, RN, ANP-BC
Guest Editor

"Illness is the night side of life, a more onerous citizenship. Everyone who is born holds dual citizenship in the kingdom of the well and in the kingdom of the sick. Although we all prefer to use only the good passport, sooner or later each of us is obliged, at least for a spell, to identify ourselves as citizens of that other place."

—*Susan Sontag, Illness as Metaphor*

I wish to thank the *Nursing Clinics of North America* for the privilege of editing an issue on long-term care. Fifteen years ago I edited a Clinics issue on community that included an article on long-term care. I recall not knowing much about long-term care. The social contexts of illness and aging were very different at that time. There were no aging baby boomers driving the demographics in a changing society. There was no economic crisis. In the 1990s, long-term care would not become a focal point for any analysis of the health care system. In 2009, it is a new millennium. Understanding long-term care is foremost in the curricula of medical and nursing students and is at the top of the list in policy think tanks. In 1998, I became an adult nurse practitioner in long-term care. I have been witness to the unfolding of a new paradigm. As chronic illness and longer life spans have changed the faces of aging, so have a broad array of issues around quality of life and illness at the end of life.

By profession, I am a nurse educator. Advanced practice with nursing home residents is my passion. I am grateful for the opportunity to integrate into this issue some of the important issues driving long-term care in the twenty-first century. Long-term care is a continuum that crosses many age groups, illnesses, and settings. It is chronic illness and a series of exacerbations and remissions in men, women, and children of all ages and any setting. Long-term care is old age, relentless in the toll it takes on the frail. It is children who live with chronic illness and lifelong disability. Long-term care is a journey rather than a series of discrete events.

The focus of this issue is on long-term care and older adults in the community and in nursing homes. Some of the articles focus on the general community and others on the nursing home. My initial objective in putting together a sequence of articles on older adults was to elucidate the issues, raise questions, and diminish the stigma that becomes part of one's identity in chronic illness. A second objective was to integrate

Nurs Clin N Am 44 (2009) xi–xiii
doi:10.1016/j.cnur.2009.03.004
0029-6465/09/$ – see front matter © 2009 Elsevier Inc. All rights reserved.

nursing.theclinics.com

the "voices" of diverse experts in the field of aging and long-term care. A third objective was to build the concept of "community" into all long-term care settings. Long-term care is an example of Susan Sontag's "other place."

I am fortunate to have best practice contributors to this issue—a physician from the reknowned Cleveland Clinic, a home care nurse executive who is director of a home and hospice organization and home care nurses, a hospital chaplain, a nursing professor emeritus, a senior nurse researcher working for the AARP in Washington, a journalist who has dedicated her work to Alzheimer's caregivers, a former inaugural fellow who recently left Washington to return to teaching at the University of Kentucky in Louisville, and a geriatrician who is an expert in palliative and hospice care. All bring a deep and tireless commitment to the care of older adults. I extend my thanks to each contributor for the thoughtful articles and good work. I also thank Clinics Editor Katie Hartner for her patience and kindness. Finally, my deep appreciation and thanks go to Bettina Elliott, my assistant for the Clinics project. Your expertise and support have been invaluable for many years.

This issue covers a lot of territory. It is always difficult to make choices about what to include in a journal with finite pages. This issue can best be described as eclectic. It has gone through many adaptations over the past 6 months. The contributors address some of the many challenges to long-term care in the twenty-first century. Part I presents an overview of the broad societal issues that significantly influence the directions of long-term care. In their discussion of the nursing workforce, Drs. Susan Reinhard and Heather Young present an articulate and informative overview of issues such as the nursing shortage, the aging of the population, the aging of practicing nurses, the aging of nurse educators, and the new demographics that so much influence all older adults. A second article analyzes the nursing workforce from a different perspective by describing the nursing shortage and concerns about long-term care, recruiting, and retaining diverse and underrepresented nursing students to the profession. Two programs are described that have been supported by HRSA grants since 2003. A compelling challenge to nursing and to health care is how to remedy the shortage of diverse registered nurses in nursing homes and how to graduate more underrepresented nurses with baccalaureate degrees who will bring us closer to addressing long-term care disparities and look forward to working in nursing home settings. A third article focuses on a discussion of long-term care disparities by Dr. Barbara Messinger-Rapport. She brings real life to the numbers through cases and strong detail. Until now, there has been limited discussion of the financial, social, and treatment inequities in nursing homes.

Part II addresses some of the clinical challenges in long-term care, keeping the focus on nursing homes. The first article by Drs. Messinger-Rapport and Dumas is an epidemiologic discussion of resident falls in nursing homes including causes, interventions, and outcomes. The second article by Drs. Dumas and Ramadurai overviews clinical problems through case analyses in the most vulnerable elderly nursing home residents. The final two articles are the "voices" of advocates, of caregivers, and of a hospital chaplain who worked in hospice for a long time. There is a spirituality in the voice of Reverend Beth Loomis as she overviews the difficult choices that families and patients must make. She guides the families through the darkest of times. The caregiver voices are those of two women, one the daughter and the second the wife of a person with advanced Alzheimer's disease. The stories of their journeys with loved ones are compelling.

In Part III, Meg Doherty, a nurse executive director of a successful home care and hospice association, describes and analyzes the organizational challenges these organizations face as long-term care becomes a dominant force in a broken health care system. A second article in this section is written by Dr. Fran Portnoy, a sociologist professor and expert in long-term care. She writes of her family through the generations as they face the challenges of aging. Now retired, she writes poignantly of the life changing experiences that accompany growing old. Drs. Susan Reinhard and Karen Robinson conclude Part III by looking ahead to the next 50 years. They write of the need for "more effective chronic care and more humane long-term care." This is a timely article in the midst of economic and social crises that are unparalleled in history.

In 2009, the state of the economy, foreclosures, huge bailouts, and devastating job losses demand all of Washington's attention. Emergency measures by Congress affect families of the chronically ill who are young and old. Nursing homes and other care facilities are affected as budgets and staff are cut. The problems in our nation divert attention from a health care system that needs to be fixed. We will continue to promote advocacy and change and humane policies. We will look to nursing leadership in chronic care as we have never before.

Again, I thank the diverse contributors to this work. I hope readers complete their reading of this Clinics issue on long-term care with a better understanding of the connections or links between the institutions and the patients, the residents, the health care providers, and all others who advocate for the vulnerable populations who profile the many faces of chronic illness, people who are "citizens of that other place."

Linda G. Dumas, PhD, RN, ANP-BC
College of Nursing and Health Sciences
University of Massachusetts Boston
100 Morrissey Boulevard
Boston, MA 02125

E-mail address:
linda.dumas@umb.edu (L.G. Dumas)

The Nursing Workforce in Long-Term Care

Susan C. Reinhard, PhD, RN, FAAN[a],*, Heather M. Young, PhD, RN, FAAN[b]

KEYWORDS

• Long-term care • Nursing workforce • Nurse delegation
• Long-term care consumers • Policy

OVERVIEW

Many—if not most—nurses think of nursing homes when they hear "long-term care" (LTC). That is because most people do the same. However, research reveals that most people do not want to go to a nursing home,[1] at least not as these institutions exist today. People prefer services and supports that help them stay in their own homes for as long as possible.

Policymakers are reinforcing this shift toward home- and community-based care as the predominant model of LTC. For example, in collaboration with state Medicaid offices, the Centers for Medicare and Medicaid Services launched the $1.75 billion "Money Follows the Person" initiative to relocate people who have been in nursing homes for at least 6 months. The US Administration on Aging developed the "Choices for Independence" initiative to divert people from nursing homes and keep more people who need long-term services in their homes. State efforts to "balance" LTC financing between institutional and home care,[2] and "global budgets" designed to provide more flexible LTC funding,[3] reinforce this direction away from nursing homes to home-based care.

As policy and financing follow consumer demand for change, nurses need to revision the future of LTC and their role in it. The call for greater nursing leadership to improve the quality of care in nursing homes is compelling.[4] However, the need for nurses to develop a more collaborative role with consumers to support community living is also pressing,[5] particularly because many consumer advocates view nurses as obstacles to their right to live outside of institutions (R. Kafka, personal communication, 2008).

This article describes the LTC nursing workforce, consumers' needs for LTC, and forces shaping future demand. It serves as a foundation for progressive thought and action to make a broader view of LTC real for all of us.

[a] AARP Public Policy Institute, Center to Champion Nursing in America, 601 E Street, NW, WA 20049, USA
[b] Betty Irene Moore School of Nursing, UC Davis Health System, 4610 X Street, Suite 4202, Sacramento, CA 95817, USA
* Corresponding author.
E-mail address: sreinhard@aarp.org (S.C. Reinhard).

Nurs Clin N Am 44 (2009) 161–168
doi:10.1016/j.cnur.2009.02.006
0029-6465/09/$ – see front matter © 2009 Elsevier Inc. All rights reserved.

nursing.theclinics.com

LTC WORKFORCE TODAY

People who need ongoing services and supports to help them with personal care, daily living activities, and chronic care turn to families, paraprofessionals, and professionals—in that order. About 80% to 90% of care recipients rely on assistance from informal caregivers.[6] Nearly 44 million family caregivers serve as the backbone of LTC, providing $350 billion in "free care."[7] These caregivers provide long-term assistance with essential daily activities, such as bathing and transferring, and about half of them perform nursing-oriented tasks, such as helping with wound care, injections, equipment, or medication administration.[8]

We often ask these family caregivers to do things that would make nursing students tremble.[9] Despite this hands-on role, family caregivers report a serious lack of communication with health care providers, inadequate training to use medical technologies and administer necessary treatments, and isolation and emotional strain associated with the need to engage in constant vigilance.[10] Family caregivers often report that doctors, nurses, social workers, and other professionals do not communicate with them, even when these same caregivers are expected to give medications, recognize and manage symptoms, perform complicated treatments, and navigate the health and long-term health and social services maze.[11]

Following family caregivers, the workforce most likely to provide LTC services are known as "paraprofessionals," which includes personal care attendants, home health aides, nursing aides, and independent providers hired directly by consumers. Estimating the size of this workforce is difficult, but the Institute for the Future of Aging Services[12] reports about 2.5 million direct care workers in both the health and LTC sectors. About half are racial or ethnic minorities, mainly women (about 90%). The Paraprofessional Health care Institute reports that by 2016, we will need a total of 4 million direct care workers.[13] This market demand for paraprofessionals is increasing attention to the need to improve salaries and benefits to make these jobs competitive enough to attract a qualified and stable direct care workforce.

There are about 500,000 registered nurses (RNs) and licensed practical nurses (LPNs) practicing in LTC, including home care, assisted living, and nursing homes[12]; almost half are LPNs. About 90% of RNs are white; the LPN workforce is more diverse. There are an unknown number of advanced practice nurses (APNs), such as nurse practitioners, working in LTC. Importantly, in addition to a shortage, the nursing workforce in LTC also lacks adequate preparation in gerontological nursing, with only 1% of all RNs and 3% of all nurse practitioners certified in geriatrics, despite the fact that most of the health care consumers are older adults.[14]

The Institute of Medicine projects the need for 3.5 million more health care workers by 2030—including 868,000 RNs and 231,000 LPNs.[15] To meet the needs of an aging country, each worker's knowledge and skills must be used as efficiently as possible with more flexible roles that we are accustomed to seeing today. To better understand the need to reshape our LTC workforce, we need to consider what consumers will need.

CONSUMERS' NEEDS FOR LTC: FORCES SHAPING FUTURE DEMAND

The population profile of the United States will change dramatically in the next 25 years, shifting toward a higher proportion of older adults and greater cultural and ethnic diversity. Both the total number of older adults and the proportion are increasing, from 12.9% of the population in 2005 to 20% in 2030. Those older than 85 years of age are the fastest growing segment of the population, expected to reach 31 million in 2050,[16] and are the most likely to be represented as consumers of health care in all settings. Minority elders will increase by 328% for Hispanics, 285% for Asian and Pacific Islanders, 147% for American Indians and Aleuts, and 131% for African Americans, compared with 81% for Caucasians, enhancing the diversity of history and values in our communities.[17] Our society will include more older adults at a time when the relative proportion of younger members is decreasing, with staggering implications for both family and formal care systems.

Over the past few decades, life expectancy has increased significantly, so that more and more older adults are living to advanced age. Although most of them remain functionally independent until age 85 years, most older adults develop chronic conditions that eventually precipitate the need for some assistance. Indeed, almost 125 million people in the United States have a chronic condition,[18] a number that is projected to rise to 158 million by 2040.[19] For persons older than 70 years of age, more than 80% have at least 1 chronic physical illness, and many have multiple chronic conditions.[20] By age 80 years, 70% of women and 53% of men experience 2 or more chronic conditions.[21] The most common chronic illnesses among those 75 years of age and older include hypertension (52.8%), heart disease (36.6%), diabetes (25%), and cancer (23.9%).[20] The trend of increasing prevalence of chronic conditions is expected to continue as both the number and proportion of older adults increase with the aging of the baby boomers.

Chronic conditions are important to consider, because they usually involve a long-term trajectory, including both acute and long-term health care needs. A number of chronic conditions, such as arthritis and heart disease, can have a significant impact on functional ability and the capacity to manage activities of daily living independently.[22] Functional impairment and frailty have implications for individuals, families, and society.[23] The increased need for both informal assistance and health care services affects lives of both those needing care and their family members.[24,25] General health is affected as those with chronic conditions report poorer physical and mental health than the general population.[24] Medical costs related to chronic illness were $470 billion in 1995 and may go as high as $864 billion by 2040.[19]

One rough indicator of the workforce supply to care for older adults is the dependency ratio, capturing the number of older adults (defined as >65 years, and, therefore, "dependent") in relation to the number of younger adults (defined as 20–64, and, therefore, "productive") in the population. This ratio has grown from 9.1 older adults per 100 workers in 1930 to 20.5 in 2000 and is projected to reach 35.7 in 2030.[16] The number of younger adults is significant for 3 main reasons: as providers of family care; as a source of workers for the geriatric workforce; and as contributors to social security. However, the calculation of the dependency ratio has been challenged, because it assumes that all members of the population between 20 and 64 years of age are productive and all of those older than 65 years of age are dependent, when in fact, many older adults are actually providing family care and many do not require functional assistance. If the dependency ratio is recalculated using age 75 years as the cutoff between productivity and dependency, the ratio actually improves between 1960 and 2030.[26]

As indicated above, the majority of LTC is provided by families, a service to society that reduces the demand on formal care systems. Yet in the coming years, the availability of family to care for older adults is expected to decline. There is a higher proportion of female-headed households and employed women,[27] reducing the number of women remaining at home. Based on the declining fertility rate and a higher proportion of childless women in the 40- to 45-year age group, there will be fewer adult children available for tomorrow's elders. Divorce rates are higher, reducing the available pool further.[28] A decline in informal care was observed during the last decade of 1900 from

70.5% to 65.8%, along with an increase in formal care from 48.7% to 59.9% among a large national sample,[29] suggesting that the demographic trends have already begun to have an effect on demand for formal care.

This increased demand for formal care could be offset by improvements in the health and functional status of older adults, particularly by modifying risk factors and health promotion efforts.[26] Authors disagree on whether improvements in health are enough to reduce demand for services. The National Long-Term Care Study reported that the disability rate for all adults older than 65 years of age declined from 26.2% in 1982 to 19.7% in 1999. Even though the population of older adults increased during this time period, there remained a net reduction of 100,000 disabled elderly in the United States.[26] On the other side, the major improvements noted in the National Long-Term Care Study were in the area of instrumental activities of daily living and do not reflect the more intensive needs of those requiring assistance with basic activities of daily living.[29]

NURSING ROLE IN LTC DELIVERY

As more older adults and people with disabilities choose to remain in their homes and communities with long-term supportive services, they are seeking practical help in managing "health-related" tasks, such as taking medications, managing daily bowel and bladder routines, and obtaining nutrition with technological support. With increasing costs of nursing homes and consumer preferences for less-restrictive environments, many states have increased the support of community-based alternatives to nursing homes. This shift from institutions, where care is organized around the 24-hour availability of staff, to community settings, where formal care is episodic, has required changes in the ways RNs deliver professional oversight and direct care for consumers.

The development and funding of nurse delegation has been an important advancement in consumer-centered care. Although delegation has always been a part of the nurse practice act in most states,[30] the practice has not always been promoted in community-based settings nor reimbursed by state funding. In 1996, Washington State introduced legislation to promote community-based alternatives, including the funding of nurse delegation in assisted living and adult foster homes. An evaluation study demonstrated improved consumer outcomes with this approach and no negative implications for safety. Communication about care improved among the team and with the consumer and family, and direct care workers reported increased satisfaction related to the training and support they received from the delegating RN. Consumers particularly valued having a choice in the setting as well as the convenience of organizing care around their own needs, rather than staff schedules. In essence, nurse delegation brought unlicensed practice under nursing supervision and provided the reimbursement and supervisory mechanisms for RN involvement in community settings.[31,32] Based on national research and dialogue with both nurses and consumers, several principles can guide the nurses' collaboration with people who want to live in their homes and communities.[5] First, nursing practice is grounded in a philosophy of collaboration with the consumer:

- Nurses emphasize strengths and abilities as they collaborate with consumers in developing individualized plans for care and supportive services.
- Nurses work with and through others (consumers, informal carers, and paid attendants/caregivers) to implement these individualized plans.
- Nurses support consumers' informed decision making and personal responsibility as consumers balance their desire for both independence and personal safety.

- Nurses have the responsibility to learn and fulfill this teaching role.
- Second, consumer self-direction principles are consistent with nursing science, practice, and ethics. These principles hold that
- Consumers have the right to pursue community living, regardless of their age or disability. This right is assured by federal law.
- Consumers may desire to direct their own care.
- Consumers may seek consultation from professionals who have the knowledge and skills to provide such consultation.

Based on these principles, and in accordance with federal law and professional ethics, the professional nurse should strive to assist the consumer to achieve the most integrated setting and least restrictive environment throughout the lifespan.

Another important arena for nursing action is around transitions in care, a priority for improvement in quality and safety for older adults.[33–35] Our health care system functions as a series of silos with teams engaged in care within and little attention to the communication and crucial handoffs between settings and providers. For example, an older adult who fractures a hip at home might experience a series of providers and settings in the coming weeks, from the emergency department at a hospital, to surgery, to a postoperative hospital unit, to a subacute rehabilitation unit, to a skilled nursing facility, and then back to home with various supports (professional and direct care workers). Each provider in this series may have a different goal and approach and commonly begins by collecting data, developing a plan, and implementing the plan.

Under our current systems, there is little emphasis on seeking information from the previous setting nor on conveying key information to the subsequent providers. The consumer and family experience discontinuity, confusion, lack of timely information, and risks to safety. Medication management across settings has received the most attention, yet other care issues also affect quality and continuity, including management of symptoms, mobilization of appropriate assistive devices, communication about necessary follow-up, and resolution of consumer concerns and questions. Nurses are present in each of these various settings and as such could serve as the "connectors" or "integrators" across the silos of care that exist, improving communication and enhancing the capacity of the overall system to manage complex health conditions across settings and over time.

SUMMARY

Over the past decade, many states have expanded community-based options and promoted the role of RNs in delegating nursing tasks to unlicensed care providers.[36–38] It is clear that nurses play a crucial role in the delivery of LTC in homes and community settings, yet full enactment of this role has not been attained. Two actions would advance this approach. First, reimbursement policies and regulations of practice in community-based settings should be updated in states where nurse delegation is lagging. Second, educational programs must emphasize this aspect of the nursing role, including how to work with and through others (direct care workers, family members) to deliver high-quality and consumer-centered care and how to manage chronic illness and functional impairment from a community-based perspective, optimizing health and self-care abilities.

Nurses and social workers can better support family caregivers by mastering knowledge and competencies.[39] Because most of the health care consumers are older adults, preparation in gerontological nursing should be foundational in all nursing programs and at every level of practice. A number of core general competencies are required for the future, including leadership in nursing and health care, collaboration with the health care team, sound clinical judgment, effective communication, relationship-based care, and appropriate use of evidence for practice.[40] Leadership is a core competency, and nurses are in a pivotal position to lead in community-based LTC by virtue of their professional expertise, their relationships with consumers, their understanding of systems issues, and their ability to work through others.[41]

APNs are ideally suited to manage the primary health care needs of community-based older adults, integrating consumer preferences and values into a plan of care that addresses health, functional, social, and emotional priorities while managing chronic illnesses and planning for end of life.[42] Post-master's educational programs are needed to ensure that all APNs have competencies in the care of older adults. With the recent change in reimbursement for home visits, a new opportunity exists for community-based APNs to deliver consumer-centered care to homebound older adults.

The nursing shortage is commonly discussed in terms of the diminishing "supply" of nurses. Another important factor in the shortage is the "demand." Because nursing expertise (RN and APN) is a precious resource, strategies to optimize the contributions of nurses are required. Demand could be reduced through work redesign in examining team approaches that ensure that the RN or APN can devote the most time and attention to those areas where their particular skills are needed, and other members of the team, including direct care workers, are included to manage the nonprofessional aspects of the role. Technology could improve the efficiency of care and access to needed information to make clinical decisions. For example, home telehealth monitoring could provide health data, such as vital signs, digital images of wounds, and information about patterns of activity, including taking medications, enabling an RN to manage care remotely in addition to in-person visits. Electronic health records accessible across settings could increase the accuracy of clinical information as well as reduce the time required to re-collect data with every encounter.

Nursing care in the future must emphasize support for family members who provide care, chronic disease management across settings and between usual health care encounters, targeted interventions to improve function and health, and sensitivity to the cultural and ethnic diversity of the population.[23] Several areas must be addressed to ensure full enactment of the nursing role: educational preparation, work redesign, and policy change.

REFERENCES

1. AARP. Fixing to Stay. Washington, DC: AARP; 2000.
2. Kassner E, Reinhard S, Fox-Grge W, et al. A balancing act: state long-term care reform. Public Policy Institute: Washington, DC: AARP; 2008.
3. Hendrickson L, Reinhard S. Global budgeting: promoting flexible funding to support long-term care choice. Rutgers Center for State Health Policy & National Academy for State Health Policy. New Brunswick (NJ): Community Living Exchange; 2004.
4. Horvath T, Swafford K, Smith K, et al. Enhancing nursing leadership in long-term care: a review of the literature. Research in Gerontological Nursing 2008;1(3).
5. Reinhard S, Young H. Guiding principles for the nurse-consumer relationship: improved collaboration and support of consumers' community living. New Brunswick (NJ): Rutgers Center for State Health Policy; 2006.
6. Spillman B, Black K. Staying the course: trends in family caregiving. Public Policy Institute. Washington, DC: AARP; 2005.

7. Gibson A, Houser K. Valuing the invaluable: a new look at the economic value of family caregiving. Washington, DC: AARP Public Policy Institute; 2007.
8. Wolff J, Kasper J. Caregiver of frail elders: updating a national profile. Gerontologist 2006;46:344–56.
9. Reinhard S. Wanted: nurses who support caregivers. Am J Nurs 2006;106(8):13.
10. Reinhard S, Huhtula N, Given B, et al. Supporting family caregivers. In: Hughes R, editor. Patient safety and quality: an evidence-based handbook for nurses. Rockville (MD): Agency for Healthcare Research and Quality; 2008. p. 1–64.
11. Levine C, Reinhard SC, Feinburg LF, et al. Family caregivers on the job: moving beyond ADLs and IADLs. Generations 2004;27:17–23.
12. Institute for the Future of Aging Services. The long-term care workforce: can the crisis be fixed? A Report prepared for the National Commission for Quality Long-Term Care. Washington, DC: Institute for the Future of Aging Services; 2006.
13. Paraprofessional Healthcare Institute. Occupational projections for direct-care workers, 2006–2016. Available at: http://phinational.org/issues/growing-demand/. Accessed September 27, 2008.
14. White House Conference on Aging. Geriatric Workforce Issues. 2005.
15. Institute of Medicine. Retooling for an aging America: building the health care workforce. In: Committee on the Future Health Care Workforce for Older Americans, editor. Washington, DC: The National Academies Press; 2008.
16. US Census. United States Census 2000. 2002.
17. Hayes-Bautista DE, Hsu P, Perez A, et al. The 'browning' of the graying of America: diversity in the elderly population and policy implications. Generations 2002;26(3):15–24.
18. Wu S, Green A. Projection of chronic illness prevalence and cost inflation. California: RAND Health; 2000.
19. The Robert Wood Johnson Foundation. Chronic care in America: a 21st century challenge. Princeton (NJ): Robert Wood Johnson Foundation; 1996.
20. National Center for Health Statistics. National Health Interview Survey. Public Health Services; 1999.
21. National Center for Health Statistics. National Health Interview Survey. Public Health Service; 2000.
22. Trupin L, Rice D. Health status, medical care use, and number of disabling conditions in the United States. Washington, DC: National Institute on Disability and Rehabilitation Research; 1995.
23. Young H. Challenges and solutions in care of frail older adults. Online J Issues Nurs 2003;8(2):4.
24. National Center for Health Statistics. National Health Interview Survey. Public Health Service; 1994.
25. US Bureau of the Census. 65+ in the United States. In: Current population reports, special studies. Washington, DC: U.S. Government Printing Office; 1996. p. P23–190.
26. Knickman J, Snell E. The 2030 problem: caring for the aging baby boomers. Health Serv Res 2002;37(4):849–84.
27. Jenkins C. Resource effects on access to long-term care for frail older people. J Aging Soc Policy 2001;13(4):35–52.
28. Wolf D. Population change: friend or foe of the chronic care system? Health Aff 2001;20(6):28–42.
29. Spillman B, Pezzin L. Potential and active family caregivers: changing networks and the "Sandwich Generation." Milbank Q 2000;78(3):347–74.

30. Kane R, O'Connor C, Baker M. Delegation of nursing activities: implications for patterns of long-term care. Washington, DC: AARP; 1995.
31. Young H, Sikma S. Nurse Delegation Study Research Report. 1998. Available at: http://www.doh.wa.gov/hsqa/uwstudy.doc. Accessed January 10, 2003.
32. Sikma S, Young H. Balancing freedom with risks: the experience of nursing task delegation in community based residential care settings. Nurs Outlook 2001; 49(4):193–201.
33. Nolan M, Grant G, Keady J, et al. Cognitively impaired older adults: from hospital to home. Am J Nurs 2005;105(2):52–61.
34. Naylor MD, Brooten DA, Campbell RL, et al. Transitional care of older adults hospitalized with heart failure: a randomized, controlled trial. J Am Geriatr Soc 2004;52:675–84.
35. Mezey M, Neveloff Dubler N, Ethel M, et al. What impact do setting and transitions have on the quality of life at the end of life and the quality of the dying process. Gerontologist 2002;42(14):54.
36. Reinhard S, Young J, Kane RA, et al. Final report: nurse delegation of medication administration for elders in assisted living. Baltimore (MD): American Nurses Foundation; 2003.
37. Reinhard SC, Young HM, Kane RA, et al. Nurse delegation of medication administration for older adults in assisted living. Nursing Outlook 2006;54(2):61–116.
38. Mitty EL. Assisted living and the role of nursing. Am J Nurs 2003;103(8):32–43.
39. Reinhard S, Kelly K, Brooks A. state of the science: nurses and social workers supporting family caregivers. Am J Nurs 2008;108(9).
40. Tanner C, Gubrud-Howe P, Shores L. Oregon consortium for nursing education: a response to the nursing shortage. Policy Polit Nurs Pract 2008.
41. Reinhard S, Reinhard T. Scanning the field. Future Age 2006;5(3):34–6.
42. Mitty E, Mezey M. Integrating advanced practice nurses in home care: recommendations for a teaching home care program. Nurs Health Care Perspect 1998;19(6):264–70.

Leadership in Nursing Homes—2009: Challenges for Change in Difficult Times

Linda G. Dumas, PhD, RN, ANP-BC[a],*, Carolyn Blanks, BA[b],
Victoria Palmer-Erbs, PhD, RN[a], Frances L. Portnoy, RN, MA, MS, PhD[a]

KEYWORDS

• Diverse • Leadership • Nursing education
• Nursing homes • Barriers

In 2006, then-Senator Barack Obama was the commencement speaker at the University of Massachusetts in Boston.

> *America is an unlikely place...and you can still rise to become whatever you want. Think globally, welcome diversity, empathize with others and fight for their dreams... There is more work to be done, more justice to be had, more barriers to break down...*[1]

This article is about nursing leadership, workforce diversity, and underrepresentation in nursing. It is about long-term care, specifically the nursing home, the nurses, and the certified nursing assistants (CNAs). The nursing shortage, the shortage of nurse educators, and curricular changes in the colleges and universities are *not* the focus of this work. Those are substantial issues for a second article at another time. The questions asked here are, *who* will care for the residents in nursing homes, and how will they recruit the much-needed leadership at a time of unprecedented need?

When I was asked to edit this issue of *Nursing Clinics*, we were fortunate to have Drs. Reinhard and Young accept an offer to contribute to an update on the nursing workforce in long-term care. Their focus was on the workforce in home- and community-based care. They gave an overview of the new aging demography, the work of informal caregivers, and "the long term care forces shaping future demand."[2] They write of *the projected need for 3.5 million more health care workers by 2030, including*

[a] University of Massachusetts Boston, College of Nursing and Health Sciences, Department of Nursing, 100 Morrissey Boulevard, Boston, MA 02125, USA
[b] Labor & Workforce Development, Massachusetts Senior Care Association, 2310 Washington Street, Suite 300, Newton Lower Falls, MA 02462, USA
* Corresponding author.
E-mail address: linda.dumas@umb.edu (L.G. Dumas).

Nurs Clin N Am 44 (2009) 169–178
doi:10.1016/j.cnur.2009.03.005
0029-6465/09/$ – see front matter © 2009 Elsevier Inc. All rights reserved.

almost 900,000 registered nurses (RNs)! Leadership is one of the "core competencies" that belong to nursing and one of the target areas to be addressed to ensure that nurses and nurse leaders of the future meet today's long-term care challenges.[3]

Using their article as a foundation for workforce demographics, this article takes another direction that is specific to the nursing home workforce. A primary assumption is that mentoring and training nurses for leadership roles in long-term care is our professional responsibility.

The preliminary challenge is nursing education and preparing nurses for long-term professional care. Long-term care is a broad continuum that includes home care, assisted living, and nursing homes. Long-term caregivers include licensed practical nurses (LPNs), diploma nurses, and baccalaureate nurses. Long-term care also requires speech pathologists, physical therapists, occupational therapists, and social workers for skilled services. It also includes *frontline workers,* who are the CNAs in the nursing homes and the home health aides in the communities. Because of the differences in job descriptions and skill levels, it is difficult to discuss issues about the need for baccalaureate- and master's-prepared nurse leaders in nursing homes without seeming to further stratify long-term care. With all due respect to the many competent and dedicated LPNs, one must ask, "Where are the registered nurses? and where are the university-prepared nurses?" They are represented by small numbers in the nursing homes. Nurse educators in colleges and universities have a critical role in directing nursing curricula. Nurse educators in nursing home settings have the responsibility for safe practice and adherence to quality indicators and standards. In the nursing home setting, the leadership role of faculty educators is less relevant than the role of staff educators as they focus on safety, training the trainers, quality care, and meeting standards set by the various accreditation guidelines. Nursing students who are currently in programs at colleges and universities have the *potential* to be the new generation of nurses and nurse leaders in nursing homes. Twenty percent of the US population, 72.5 million people, will be older than 65 years by 2030, with 31 million older than 85 years by 2050.[2] Another stunning statistic that supports a mandate for change is that minority elders will increase by 200% to 300%![2] Compare this to the 81% cited for Caucasians. Long-term care policy makers say that the health care system must change to meet the demands of an aging society.[4] This has been repeated for a long time.[4]

As more people in minority groups grow old and live in nursing homes, the need for registered nurses from diverse racial, ethnic, cultural, and economic backgrounds, who will better represent the residents in the nursing homes, becomes very important. The dilemma is how to recruit and retain committed nurses and a new cadre of nurse leaders to meet long-term care demands over the next 50 years. This can be done without sacrificing the commitment to diversity by taking a long and constructively critical look at workforce and nursing home disparities.

AGAIN, THE PRESIDENT'S WORDS

We want to think globally, seek diversity, help people to reach their "dreams" and continue to break down the barriers that are keeping them from doing so.[1]

Capturing diversity, "reaching dreams," and "breaking down barriers" are far reaching goals. Long-term care is a complicated specialty and the nursing home is a complex environment. Is it a medical home? Can it ever be a medical home? Is it a community? Can it be a community when there are so many residents with serious illnesses, dementias, and multiple comorbidities? Reinhard and Young talk about "the *greening* of the nursing home."[2] Would the "greening," or changing the nursing home to a community culture with smaller, more home-like environments, even be feasible? Or does the concept of greening of the nursing home more narrowly refer to a more financially accessible assisted-living model, with retirement communities, and other places, where older adults, even the very old who are healthier than their nursing home counterparts, live?[5,6] Illness, particularly chronic illness, always has a social context. Today's nursing homes are places of high acuity. There is an integration of posthospital rehab patients and long-term care residents who are also patients. Patients on long-term care are often quite ill with multiple medical issues and comorbid conditions. The short-term rehab patients are ill but are expected to recover and go home. Many of them are very ill, suffer complications, and don't leave. The acuity profiles of patients in nursing homes are changing. This is all the more reason for nursing homes to recruit RNs and baccalaureate-prepared RNs to work in them. This is also a compelling rationale for bringing educational opportunities and clinical ladder choices to the most passionate and dedicated frontline nursing home workers: the CNAs.

A new kind of nursing workforce is needed in long-term care, and specifically in the nursing homes: a workforce that is educated, that is diverse at all levels, and that comes from underrepresented groups and various cultures. As the number of elders in minority groups increases, it makes good sense to recruit nurses who are culturally competent and professionally able to represent resident needs. As nursing schools reach capacity, it should be ensured that a group of diverse students form a core group of "best students" and that they receive a consistent education in long-term care and geriatrics. Accelerated programs and online RN–to–Bachelor of Science in Nursing (BSN) programs should be accessible to these groups.

DIVERSITY IS EVERYONE'S BUSINESS

Any discussion of the nursing workforce, the nursing shortage, and the recruitment and retention of nursing students is complex. Add the long-term care setting and the nursing needs increase in complexity. First, there is a *shortage of nurses;* second, there is a *shortage of nurse educators* in the universities; third, there is *an untapped population* of high school students, nursing home CNAs, and community based individuals who are in allied health work and want to be nurses; and fourth, there is a new level of acuity in the nursing home residents.

These issues are complex. The specific shortage of nurse educators, and especially nurse educators who have an interest in long-term care, is of compelling concern. There are disparities in the nursing workforce and in patient care settings.[7] Change is here and there are new opportunities to reach out to underrepresented nursing students, home health workers, and nursing home CNAs and LPNs. It makes sense to first educate individuals who are already committed to working in nursing homes in various roles. How does one redirect baccalaureate nursing students as graduates to long-term care? How does one reach out and prepare men and women in the community who are interested in long-term care? How does one reach out to students from urban high schools to prepare for a nursing career? How does one support them, provide financial aid, and implement small learning communities, such as nursing clubs, where they gain self-confidence and direction from the safety of small groups of students who know each other? How does one change the dismal graduation rate of public schools in large urban areas? How does one connect the future, with its aging demographics, with the dreams of a new cadre of nurses and nurse leaders? *How does one fight for their dreams and break down the barriers to a university education?*

This section deals with some state-of-the-art programs that achieve the desired outcomes: developing well prepared nurses who are passionate about long-term care and bringing more RNs to nursing homes.

The nursing shortage is not going to be resolved any time soon because there are long lines of prospective students on hold because of a lack of nurse educators. One of Edmund's 8 suggestions is to develop more *nontraditional programs, technology*, and *new geriatric-based curricula*. The online RN to BSN curriculum is an example, as are the accelerated programs for qualified students and the non-nursing BSN to master's degree programs. The unfortunate reality is that few BSN graduates will move on their own to long-term care. The need is for a refocused education and mentoring. The profession needs multidisciplinary collaboration and co-ordination to implement more programs.

There are not enough educational partnerships. Nonprofit organizations such as the Massachusetts Senior Care Association need to be recognized and utilized; the profession needs more than just academia. Nurse educators, administrators, and deans are retiring and nurses with graduate education are choosing practice over teaching. There are long lines of prospective nursing students on wait lists because colleges and universities cannot accommodate the numbers. The "grim truth" about the nursing faculty shortage is that without nurse educators, the nursing crisis will only get worse.[8] The mandate for RNs and baccalaureate-prepared RNs in nursing homes must be addressed. Student nurses and new graduates have very little interest in nursing homes or long-term care. How does one address this problem in nursing curricula? How does one present the care of the old to the young future caregivers? What does one teach, and where in the curriculum does one teach geriatrics and long-term care? What does one teach nursing students about caring for the old, the sick, and the dying?

One solution is to provide opportunities to nursing assistants and LPNs in the nursing homes. Provide opportunities to prepare them to enter nursing programs. These workers, especially the CNAs, are *the frontline providers*; most are passionate about what they do, and many are men and women of color. Most never get the opportunity to become RNs. This article should be seen as a "white paper": nonprescriptive, with a discussion of demographic trends and alternative ways of looking at the long-term care problem. The reader can suggest ideas about how to change the nursing home and educate the frontline caregivers. Again, the Obama refrain: *How do we fight for their dreams?*[1] How does one integrate passion for one's work, commitment to the old, and nursing education? This "white paper" model addresses the strength of community partnerships and programs.

In 1994, Penny Hollander Feldman, a long-time champion of men and women in home care and nursing home service jobs, edited an issue of *Generations*, the journal of the American Society on Aging.[9] The issue is about the men and women who work in home care as home health aides or in nursing homes as CNAs—the "frontline workers in long-term care"[10] "It's both—roses and onions," said Elena, a nursing home CNA. "Caring for old people isn't always easy." The roses are the rewards of giving to others, making others comfortable and safe; the onions are the difficult times, the hard work, the long hours, and the lack of financial reward. It is an opportunity to care for the most frail and the most vulnerable in the health care system. It is also an opportunity to fine-tune one's impressions or perspectives on life. Caring for the sick on any level is hard, often emotionally draining work. But it is a series of everyday, routine encounters with the sick that forces providers to come to terms with life, death, and the suffering that often bridges the two.

Frontline work is "dirty work," as sociologist Everett Hughes called it.[11] It is changing diapers, cleaning after incontinence, bathing, feeding, and helping patients with the most intimate routines of daily life. "It is not for sissies."[11] RNs are no longer frontline workers in many hospitals. They have more education, increasingly complex responsibilities, and spend less time with the patients. The concept of "frontline" is directed more to the CNAs and home health workers. Many are unsung heroes!

Genevay, in her wonderful portrayal of frontline workers in nursing homes, writes:

[Being a frontline worker] is for the multitude of creative, sensitive, intelligent helpers who want to learn how to grow personally and professionally through their commitment to disabled and dying elderly.[10]

These are the qualities that are wanted in providers and skilled caregivers. Qualities of leadership and commitment are necessary when one's life work is caring for the sick, the old, and the dying. Most of these frontline workers have low salaries, marginal health benefits, and very hard working lives. Their hours are long, they are not considered professionals, and they reap few of the benefits that professionals receive. "Attracting, retaining and providing recognition for high quality CNAs is an ever present challenge facing long-term care facilities across the country."[10]

Recruiting qualified, interested CNAs to nursing school makes good sense. This is as true in 2009 as it was in 1994 when this issue of *Generations* was written. Nursing home leaders have worked hard to bring recognition and opportunity to the CNAs through clinical ladders in nursing homes. The clinical ladder is a way of transitioning frontline workers to nursing schools. Many nursing homes provide a clinical ladder reward system. The Massachusetts Senior Care Association and Carolyn Blanks have made significant inroads to transitioning CNAs to nursing schools.

DIVERSITY LEADERSHIP MODELS: BRINGING THE BEST TO NURSING AND THE NURSING SCHOLARS PROGRAMS

This section deals with a *workforce diversity program model* as a vehicle for bringing underrepresented men and women to the nursing workforce and bringing underrepresented boys and girls in the high schools to nursing careers via 2-year and 4-year colleges and universities.

A strong funding interest of the Health Resource and Services Administration (HRSA) is the promotion of diversity in the nursing workforce. The nursing workforce is in a difficult situation, first because of a looming nursing shortage over the next 20 years, and second because of a lack of underrepresented nurses. Underrepresentation means not enough nurses who are disadvantaged by race, ethnicity, disability, income, and education. *Disadvantaged* is not meant pejoratively. The bottom line is that the nursing workforce does not represent the populations being served. HRSA has awarded 2 well-funded 3-year grants to the University of Massachusetts Boston. The first grant was to model a program called Bringing the Best to Nursing (BBN). The grant ran from 2003 to 2006 and 130 underrepresented men and women were accepted. The second program is currently in place and funded from 2007 to 2010. This program is built on lessons learned from the BBN program. It is called the Nursing Scholars Program (NSP). The program relies on a collaborative effort of multiple communities, including the university, neighborhoods, schools, and health care institutions. It is teaching the profession important lessons about recruiting and retaining minority students in nursing. The model has the challenge of directing the students to long-term care scholarships, frontline work while in school, and ultimately a career in caring for the old in nursing home settings.

COMPELLING PORTRAITS OF DIVERSITY

The nursing shortage involves much more than the number of workers. There is also a shortage of minority and other underrepresented populations already in the workforce. This means that in Massachusetts and many other states, the workforce will not mirror the population it is meant to serve. Why is this important? It is increasingly relevant that cultural and ethnic groups are not represented in professional roles and that community groups do not have the advocacy of nurses who understand their issues. These pressing concerns are what shaped the BBN and the NSP programs.

Why is all this information relevant to long-term care and this issue of *Clinics*? Because long-term care, in particular nursing home care, is mostly staffed by LPNs and CNAs. There is opportunity to offer education and training for the RN role. Clinical ladder programs at individual nursing homes are expensive, and in these economic times, there are fewer opportunities available for higher education.

The diversity programs are based on a culture of community model. Community is the foundation of the programs. A *culture of community model* involves diverse community and college program faculty as advisors, peer facilitators, and guest speakers for "hot topics in nursing" seminars. They are student advocates and have strong support systems. Community is viewed as a sacred place, a place where one feels safe; where the student trusts that the program is in his/her best interest. The concept of "community" runs through the NSP just as it did for the BBN groups a few years ago. The students increasingly understand the meaning of community as they move through the 3-semester program.

Creating a community of students means that what each student does is everyone's business. The focus is always on the student. Students feel cared about and self-esteem rises as they are taught entry level leadership skills through stress management and resiliency seminars, English as a second language (ESL) workshops, and peer groups. The concept of a "community culture" is an important one and the outcome data reflect that the programs are making a difference in students' lives.

> I will remain ever grateful… thank you so much for taking the time to put a humane touch on what you do.
> I want to thank you for believing in me…. Your support has been priceless… with the program I learned not only how to become a nurse but also how to be a good human being.
> Your BBN grant program has given me leadership and management skills to make me a more well-rounded clinician.

One of our partnerships has been with the Massachusetts Senior Foundation, which mentors and funds underrepresented students. It is a community partnership that is being highlighted as a vehicle, promoting access to higher education and building a road to long-term care nursing for students. The following section discusses the Massachusetts Senior Association. My colleague, Carolyn Blanks, writes of the work she does with the long term-care workforce, diversity, and directors of nursing in nursing homes. This is a preliminary article and there are no quick answers. It is a "white paper" of sorts, a reflection, a vehicle for sharing ideas, personal experiences, and ways to better connect the frontline workers to the college nursing programs.

COMMUNITY PARTNERSHIPS FOR DIVERSITY—A DOOR TO NURSING FOR IMMIGRANTS

The Massachusetts Senior Care Association (Mass Senior Care) is the trade association for more than 500 nursing and rehabilitation facilities, assisted-living residences, continuing care retirement communities, and other organizations that provide health care for older adults and persons with disabilities. Since its founding in 1949, Mass Senior Care's mission has been to improve the quality and delivery of long-term care services in Massachusetts *through advocacy and education*. Workforce development is a key component of ensuring quality care, and Mass Senior Care has taken a lead role in developing strategies and facilitating partnerships to address the nursing staff shortage in long-term care.

Over the past 23 years, the Mass Senior Care Foundation, the nonprofit education and research arm of Mass Senior Care, has distributed over $2 million in scholarships to more than 1,600 long-term care employees. The program is funded through donations by Mass Senior Care members. Most of the awardees are CNAs, the frontline workers spoken about in this article. They are qualified and passionate about pursuing a nursing degree. Long-term care has become a gateway of employment for immigrants, and the increasing diversity of scholarship recipients—more than one-third of last year's awardees were immigrants and/or ethnic minorities. They are, in turn, slowly helping to diversify a predominantly white licensed nursing workforce. Many former scholarship winners who began as CNAs have not only stayed in long-term care but have advanced their nursing education to assume positions of leadership in their organizations. Donna's story is a wonderful example of a CNA who is now an RN in long-term care. She *makes a difference* because she wants to be there.

Donna Campbell, a 2-time Foundation Scholarship winner, exemplifies the difficult and circuitous path that low-income long-term care workers must successfully navigate to obtain a nursing degree. A Jamaican immigrant, Donna came to this country as a young teenager, and she had to drop out of high school to care for her siblings while her mother worked. Her first job was as a personal care assistant to an elderly couple; she later obtained her CNA certification to work at a local nursing facility. Once there, she began the road to achieving her "lifelong goal of becoming an RN certified in gerontology" by obtaining her high school equivalency, and with the support of her employer and the scholarship award, she enrolled in a community college where she graduated as an LPN. She received her second scholarship in 2008, and is now on her way to completing her RN degree while working full time at the Julian Leavitt Family Nursing Home in Longmeadow, Massachusetts. She is a leader on her unit and has successfully encouraged her peers to follow her example and enroll in RN programs.

A PARTNERSHIP TO IMPROVE CNA RETENTION IN NURSING HOMES; BRIDGES TO NURSING—INVESTING IN CNAS

Long-term care employers recognize the value of investing in their employees who are *already* passionate about their elderly patients and committed to working in a long-term care setting. Career ladders have become an integral component of the development of the Massachusetts long-term care nursing workforce. In response to a critical CNA shortage in the late 1990s, Mass Senior Care partnered with the Boston Private Industry Council to develop and pilot a 3-tiered career ladder to improve CNA retention under a 2-year federal grant. That project resulted in reduced turnover and improved wages for participating CNAs and subsequently became the model for a statewide "Extended Care Career Ladder Initiative (ECCLI)," the centerpiece of a broader state legislative initiative to improve the quality of nursing home care.

Managed by the Commonwealth Corporation, a quasi-public organization under the Massachusetts Office of Labor and Workforce Development, ECCLI provides grants to nursing facility and home care employers to support the development of career ladders, education, and skills training for CNAs and other entry level workers. With employer coinvestment, ECCLI also funds "wraparound" programs and services to meet the needs of career ladder participants, including adult basic education, English for speakers of other languages (ESOL), career counseling, communication, mentorship and leadership training, and "bridge to nursing" programs.

Since 2001, more than 170 long-term care employers, including nearly one-third of Massachusetts nursing homes, have implemented career ladder programs, resulting in new skills, opportunities for advancement, and increased wages for more than 7,500 workers. Other benefits have included improved communication, teamwork, and mutual respect among frontline staff, nurses, clients, and their families, enabling better relationships and a higher quality of care.[3,12,13]

Many CNAs who have benefited from ECCLI want to further their nursing education. Mass Senior Care has helped its members pursue a "grow their own nurses" strategy through identifying potential funding resources and partnerships. To date, more than 60 nursing homes have developed proprietary LPN programs for their staff in partnership with area community colleges or other nursing programs. Employers provide tuition, flexible work schedules, continuation of benefits, tutoring, and mentoring. Although the process may take longer than hoped for, the student graduation rate of these customized, employer-supported programs is typically higher than the rate of the general nursing student population, enabling CNAs, many of whom are from diverse and/or disadvantaged backgrounds, to receive a nursing education. Some employers are now developing LPN to RN programs to better meet the care needs of an increasingly frailer and medically complex patient population.

Since 2001, the success of ECCLI "grow your own nursing programs," the Foundation Scholarship program, and a state-funded "Direct Care Worker Training Program," administered by Mass Senior Care to provide free CNA training to people interested in entering a career in long-term care, have collectively helped to stabilize CNA vacancy rates from 15% to 8%.[3] Nearly three-fourths of all nursing staff have been employed at the same facility for 1 year or longer. Yet there are nearly 3,700 nursing staff openings in nursing homes across the state—with 1 out of every 6 RN positions vacant. (Mass Senior Care Nursing Facility Employment Survey, November 2008) This shortage will increase exponentially given the heightened demand for health care services by an aging population.

Long-term care facilities must attract more nursing students to long-term care if they are to ever fully solve their nursing workforce shortage. In 2003, Mass Senior Care convened a Long-Term Care Nursing Shortage Group, comprising representatives from nursing schools, long-term care providers, and government agency officials, to identify and implement solutions to barriers that impeded the recruitment and retention of nurses in long-term care and to educate nursing students. A key recommendation of this group is that all nursing students should be exposed to geriatrics through their academic and clinical experiences, so that they are more likely to consider working in senior care and are better prepared to care for older adult patients, regardless of setting. On April 5, 2009, Mass Senior Care will host 1,300 nursing students and faculty from programs across Massachusetts at its fifth annual Long-Term Care Nursing Day. The purpose of this popular event is to educate nursing students—and the faculty who guide them—about the rewarding careers and opportunities for nurses who work in long-term care. The event includes national speakers, student and faculty workshops, a *Long-Term Care Nursing… Explore the Possibilities* video, a job fair, and transportation at no cost to the schools of nursing or students. Developed in consultation with the Long-Term Care Nursing Shortage Group, convened by Mass Senior Care, and comprised of nursing school deans, long-term care nurses, and government agency officials, Long-Term Care Nursing Day has been an effective tool to positively shift attitudes or misconceptions that students and faculty often have about working in long-term care. In fact, two-thirds of students surveyed who opposed working in long term-care prior to the event indicated that they would now consider it an option. One said, "… It made me realize the benefits of working in long-term care and how you can make a difference in someone's life."

In the coming year, Mass Senior Care will be collaborating with its partners to increase the number of long-term care clinical sites and ensure that these clinical experiences are positive for students, faculty, and facilities. Mass Senior Care recognizes that much work remains to be done on the part of the long-term care community to provide a working environment that supports and mentors new nurses and offers continued opportunities for professional advancement and commensurate compensation. Adequate Medicaid reimbursement and funding for nursing education and ESOL are critical to ensure the continuation of career ladder and other nursing education initiatives that have effectively helped to expand the scope, skills, and diversity of the long-term care nursing workforce.

SUMMARY

Yes, this is America—a changing America. A new era is being ushered in by an African American president. This gives all of us hope for better futures; it gives those with less hope an opportunity to establish a place, one's *very own place*, in that future. There is a new focus on public and community service and on helping others to achieve their potential. The goal for nursing homes is to support residents by investing in nurses who look like the populations they serve; it is a goal to make college a reality to frontline workers in long-term care. It is a goal to bring to the nursing workforce not just diverse, but college educated, nurses. Most importantly, by choice, all of these men and women have a deep commitment to the work they do. This is our dream. That is the dream of many frontline workers and underrepresented nursing students. Leadership becomes a real option for them—they are being trained to develop that personal strength. And this is America! What a way to integrate a love for service with the RN role.

FURTHER READINGS

Aldebron A. A systematic assessment of strategies to address the nursing faculty shortage. Nurs Outlook 2008;56:286–97.

Buerhous PL, Donelan K, Ulrich B, et al. State of the registered nurse workforce in the United States. Nurs Econ 2006;24(1):6–12.

Christmas K, Close L, Estes CL, et al. A political economy perspective on frontline workers in long term care. Generations Journal of the American Society on Aging 1994;18(3):23–7.

Downs FC. The servant-leadership worldview. Annals of Long-Term Care Nursing 2007;15(8).

Dumas L, Trevens T, Ressler P. Promoting workforce diversity on an urban campus. Teaching transformation. Hum Architect J Sociol Self Knowl 2008;V1(1):53–60.

Dumas L. Bringing the best to nursing. On Call Magazine 2005;23–5.

Feldman PH, Sapienza AM, Kane NM. On the home front. The job of the home aide. Frontline workers in long term care. Generations Journal of the American Society on Aging 1994;18(3):16–9.

Harvath TA, Swafford K, Smith KML, et al. Enhancing nursing leadership in long term care: a review of the literature. Research in Gerontological Nursing 2008;1(3): 187–96.

Heineman J, Wasko M. Institute for the Future of Aging Services, American Association of Homes and Services for the Aging. Gottlieb A, Wilson K (Gerontology Institute, University of Massachusetts Boston). The qualitative evaluation of ECCLI. Commonwealth Corporation Research and Evaluation 2008; 5(2).

Henderson N. Bed, body, and soul. The job of the nursing home aide. Frontline workers in long term care. Journal of the American Society on Aging 1994; 18(3):20–2.

Karnes J, Atchley RC. Usual organizational practices in Ohio. Oxford (OH): Scripps Gerontology Center, Miami University; 1999.

Massachusetts Extended Care Federation. 2000 Employment trends in Massachusetts nursing facilities. Massachusetts Extended Care; 2000. p. 29–30.

Massachusetts Senior Care Association. 2008 Employment trends in Massachusetts nursing facilities. Massachusetts Senior Care Association; 2008. p. 31–3.

Ohio Long-Term Care Research Project. Recruiting and retaining frontline workers in long term care. Oxford (OH): Scripps Gerontology Center, Miami University; 1999.

Valentine S. Nursing leadership and the new nurse. Available at: http://juns.nursing.arizona.edu/articlesFall2002. Accessed March 14, 2009.

REFERENCES

1. Obama B. University of Massachusetts, Boston: a commencement to remember [keynote address]; 2006.
2. Reinhard S, Young H. The nursing workforce in long term care. Nurs Clin North Am 44, in press.
3. Jones R, Morris N, Singh N, et al. Improving the quality of care: a closer look. Commonwealth Corporation Research and Evaluation 2006;4(2). Available at: http://www.cbwl.org/researchandevaluation/pdf/ResearchBrief4-02.pdf.
4. Christmas K, Close L, Estes CL, et al. A political economy perspective on frontline workers in long term care. Generations American Society on Aging 2004;18(3):23–7.
5. Angelelli J. Promising models for transforming long term care. Gerontologist 2006;46(4):428–30.
6. Rabig J, Thomas W, Kane R, et al. Radical redesign of nursing homes: applying the green house concept in Tupelo, Mississippi. Gerontologist 2006;46(4):533–9.
7. Messinger-Rapport B. Disparities in long term healthcare. Nurs Clin North Am 44, in press.
8. Edmunds MW, Scudder L. The grim truth about the faculty shortage in nursing. Nursing Outlook 2006;56:286–97. Available at: http://www.medscape.com/viewarticle/586845. Accessed January 23, 2009.
9. Feldman PH. Frontline workers in long-term care. Generations Journal of the American Society on Aging 1994;18(3).
10. Genevay B. Roses and onions: the fruits of helping old and dying people. Generations Journal of the American Society on Aging 1994;18(3):13–5.
11. Hughes E. Men and their work. Westport (CT): Greenwood Press; 1981.
12. Blanks C. Staffing is education-driven. American Health Care Association Provider Magazine 2004;1:45.
13. Blanks C. Making a difference in Massachusetts. American Health Care Association Provider Magazine 2000;59–60.

Disparities in Long-Term Healthcare

Barbara Messinger-Rapport, MD, PhD, CMD, FACP

KEYWORDS

- Health disparity • Nursing home • Assisted living
- Chronic disease • End of life

The goals of Healthy People 2010 (**Fig. 1**) recognize health disparities as a barrier to providing quality of care to everyone regardless of gender, race or ethnicity, education or income, disability, geographic location, or sexual orientation.[1] Examples of health disparities affecting older adults include the much lower vaccination rate for influenza and pneumococcus in Hispanics and African Americans compared with that in whites;[2] lower rates of prescriptions for pain control in cancer-related pain for Hispanic and African Americans;[3] and lower rates of procedures for knee and hip replacements, carotid endarterectomies, and coronary-artery bypass grafting for African Americans.[4] Many aspects of the health care system may contribute to these disparities, including lack of or inadequacies in health coverage; lack of access to qualified physicians; lack of health literacy; geographic factors such as rural versus urban or region of the country.

Health disparities in the subset of approximately 1.6 million older adults residing in nursing homes is not well studied but deserves more attention, given that approximately 1 in 4 Americans spend their last days in a nursing home.[5] Disparities in the nursing home reflect both the preexisting health care disparities in the general community as well as the influence of organizational and reimbursement factors imposed by the nursing home.

This article provides a historical review of relevant demographic and financial aspects of minority usage of nursing homes and identifies health care disparities associated with long-term care. Because there is so few data on Hispanic and Asian minorities in the nursing home, most of the examples revolve around African Americans. The discussion and conclusion suggest future directions to consider to meet Healthy People 2010 goals for the frailest elders.

BACKGROUND

Before the 1960s, minorities were much less likely than their white counterparts to reside in a nursing facility. Nursing homes were typically racially segregated (by law

Section of Geriatric Medicine, Cleveland Clinic Lerner College of Medicine, Case Western Reserve University, Mail Code A91, 9500 Euclid Avenue, Cleveland, OH 44195, USA
E-mail address: rapporb@ccf.org

Nurs Clin N Am 44 (2009) 179–185
doi:10.1016/j.cnur.2009.02.005
0029-6465/09/$ – see front matter © 2009 Elsevier Inc. All rights reserved.

nursing.theclinics.com

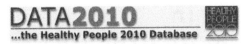

Fig. 1. Goals of Healthy People 2010: To *eliminate* health disparities and to *increase* quality and years of healthy life. (*From* Centers for Disease Control. Data 2010. Available at: http:// wonder.cdc.gov/data2010/index.htm. Accessed February 15, 2009.)

or by default), and the cost likely placed nursing homes out of reach of minorities. Minority entry into the nursing home in large numbers was likely facilitated by the introduction of Medicaid as a payer in 1966. The Medicaid program became the largest purchaser of nursing home services by the 1990s.[6] By 2004, nursing home use by blacks became 32% higher than that of whites.[7]

Despite legal elimination of segregation in 1964, nursing homes today remain relatively segregated more than 40 years later, with two-thirds of all African American residents living in just 10% of all facilities in 2000.[8] The degree of segregation varies by location, with the Midwest having the highest degree of segregation and the south having the least. African Americans are significantly more likely to be served by facilities in the bottom quartile of many structural and performance measures of quality, such as staffing, inspection deficiencies, and financial viability.[8]

Finances likely play a significant role in both the degree of segregation and the quality of care in the facility. African Americans are 30% more likely to have Medicaid as a payer source than whites.[7] Thus, nursing facilities with higher proportions of older African American residents are associated with heavy reliance on Medicaid.[8] Medicaid rates are generally less than private-pay rates and sometimes less than actual costs of care, potentially limiting resources available on-site.[9] Most homes with large proportions of African Americans are also privately owned, for-profit institutions, so they have no other source of revenue, such as philanthropy. Homes unable to attract sufficient private-pay patients tend to have lower nurse staffing levels and more serious inspection deficiencies.[10] Nursing homes that have preferential admission policies for a selective religion or continuing care community may in practice (although not on paper) be limiting first-day-elegible Medicaid admissions. This practice facilitates admissions to those with sufficient resources that they are less likely to become eligible for Medicaid during their remaining lifetime, creating mainly white, female residential population.

MANAGEMENT OF CHRONIC DISEASE

Consider an 80-year-old, long-term resident, Mrs. Carter. She is a retired African American teacher, with diabetes, atrial fibrillation, hypertension, compensated heart failure, and a history of a mild stroke 5 years ago. She exhausted her private funds 2 years ago, and Medicaid now covers the cost of her nursing home care. Despite her medical conditions, she is fairly spry and cheerful, enjoying church services, card games, news groups, and gossiping with visitors. She fell once last year, bruising her knee, but did not sustain any other injuries.

As an African American nursing home resident, she is more likely than a white resident to be hospitalized with a potentially inappropriate medication (PIM).[11] She is less likely to receive antidiabetic medications.[12] She is less likely to be prescribed Warfarin for atrial fibrillation in the setting of a prior stroke.[13] If she lives in a for-profit nursing facility, she may be more likely to be exposed to influenza, because employee vaccination rates are lower than those in nonprofit facilities.[14]

However, if she happens to be living in a facility with few African American residents, she will be less likely to be hospitalized than she would be in a facility with more African

American residents.[15] Facilities with fewer black residents typically rely less on Medicaid as a payer; they may be able to afford more staff and services and, potentially, be better able to manage chronic disease, promote an active lifestyle both physically and cognitively, and reduce hospitalization. For example, facilities that have more than 35% private-pay residents employ mid-level practitioners (nurse practitioners [NPs] or physician assistant [PA]), use intravenous (IV) therapy, or have a certified nurse aide program are less likely to hospitalize residents for acute coronary syndrome.[16]

ADDRESSING END-OF-LIFE ISSUES

End-of-life care in the nursing home is considered unsatisfactory by many residents and families. Unmet needs include addressing pain and dyspnea, physician communication, emotional support, and being treated with respect.[17]

Consider the case of Mrs. Jones, an 85-year-old African American woman with moderate to severe dementia. She was admitted to the nursing home following several hospitalizations and had recently been diagnosed with systolic heart failure, with an ejection fraction of 12%. She was prescribed 12 medications requiring more than 20 pills daily, not unusual in a person with multiple medical conditions. Despite her dementia, she can express her needs and recognize her family. She was tearful, disoriented, in pain from severe shoulder arthritis, and occasionally agitated—once taking off her clothes in the hallway and another time threatening the housekeeping staff with a table knife. She has a poor appetite and lost 20 lb in the past 6 months. Her family states that she has no advance directives, and she has always been a "full code" during hospitalizations, because they are concerned that the hospital will not offer appropriate treatment to those with a "do not resuscitate" (DNR) status.

If Mrs. Jones lives in a for-profit, primarily Medicaid facility, she is less likely to be the beneficiary of special programs, such as dementia, palliative care, or hospice.[18] Should her heart failure require IV therapy, she would need to be hospitalized, since for-profit facilities are less likely to offer specialized clinical services, such as peripherally inserted central lines, to manage heart failure.[18]

It is not unusual that Mrs. Jones has no advance directive of any type. African Americans are less likely than whites to have DNR orders[19] or living wills;[20] Hispanics are about one-third as likely as whites to have DNR orders although just as likely as whites to have living wills.[20] Since advance directives are felt to enhance autonomy and improve the quality of care at the end of life, this disparity suggests that minority residents are relatively disadvantaged.

Should Mrs. Jones continue to lose weight, she will likely be offered a feeding tube. Residents of large, for-profit, urban nursing homes with a higher percentage of nonwhite residents are more likely to have feeding tubes in the setting of severe cognitive impairment.[21] Experiences with the health care system and problems with trust in physician and nursing staff affect decisions regarding feeding tubes in dementia.[22]

DISCUSSION

Health disparities in the community likely result from the interplay of insurance; access to qualified physicians and services; health literacy and cultural disparities; and geographic distribution. Health disparities in the nursing home may be more complex because of the impact of the nature of the facility on care and care outcomes. The example of hospitalization risks provides insight into the complexity of health disparities and the interaction of underlying predictive factors. In the 2 examples of hospitalization, one by Gruneir and colleagues[15] on hospitalization and one by Intrator and colleagues[16] on hospitalization for acute coronary syndrome, simply residing in a facility with a high concentration of African Americans or Medicaid residents increases the risk of hospitalization for all residents, regardless of race or ethnicity.[15,16]

The entrance of mid-level practitioners into long-term care may improve adherence to chronic care guidelines, reduce hospital admission rates, and decrease the total number of medications.[23] For example, if there were an NP or a PA involved with Mrs. Carter's care and partnering with the physician, the burdens and benefits of anti-coagulation might have been addressed more thoroughly. The mid-level practitioner may query staff about her postural instability and the effect of potential loss of function should she have a stroke and may spend time with her and her family discussing the burden and benefit of oral anticoagulation. The result would be a more carefully crafted decision and likely closer monitoring.

Additionally, there is evidence that physicians who specialize in nursing home care are on-site at nursing homes more frequently and have quicker response times to emergencies.[24,25] The American Medical Directors Association developed a Certified Medical Director program in 1991, which includes a week-long course of didactic sessions with past training and experience. Recertification requires Continuing Medical Education in nursing home care and management. There are now nearly 2,400 Certified Medical Directors. States may begin to demand a level of geriatric education in the nursing home practitioner. The state of Maryland, in 2000, began to phase in proscriptive requirements for the education of physicians in geriatric principles to improve nursing home care in their state.[26,27]

Improving reimbursement rates of facilities from Medicaid may be helpful as well, since Medicaid often does not cover the actual cost of care in the facility. In the study by Gruneir, each $10 increment in Medicaid reimbursement reduced the odds of hospitalization by 4% for white residents and 22% for African Americans.[15] Facilities with primarily urban and minority residents are the most likely to benefit, and care could be improved by using the incremental income for staffing and additional special programs to provide higher-quality care.

Interventions in end-of-life care in the nursing home are being addressed by multiple organizations. The American Medical Directors Association has a toolkit entitled Palliative Care in the Long-Term Care Setting, to be used by medical directors and interdisciplinary teams in the nursing home. Palliative care consultations by specialists (typically a Hospice medical director or advance NP) are now reimbursable at a facility irrespective of whether the resident is receiving skilled or custodial care. For a resident active in hospice, the hospice nurses will attend an interdisciplinary care conference and help keep family members apprised of the resident's condition. The resident will receive extra attention in terms of an aide and may receive services that the facility does not have (music therapy, massage therapy, etc). The family will be monitored for complicated grieving for a year after the resident's death.

Unfortunately, interdisciplinary palliative care programs are not reimbursable by Medicare. The typical person enrolled in a palliative care program has a limited life expectancy (usually 6–12 months) or would qualify for hospice (less than a 6-month life expectancy) but refuses. Palliative care is appropriate for any stage of illness when there is a transition from treatment according to disease guidelines to meeting comfort needs, both physical and spiritual.

Mrs. Jones (details of the case have been changed to maintain privacy) was actually enrolled into a new palliative care program offered by our facility. She and her family completed a survey of their concerns and values. The family stated they did not want hospitalization because of the delirium incurred by each hospitalization, but they did not want to forgo hospitalization for worsening symptoms. Medications that did not clearly provide comfort (such as a statin) were eliminated, but medications that promoted better respiration were continued and adjusted (angiotensin-converting enzyme inhibitor, nitroglycerin). She received 3 doses of IV Lasix (Furosemide) in the facility, and then Aldactone (Spironolactone) was added to her regimen. She was given low doses of narcotics and a course of therapy for her shoulder pain, with remarkable improvement. During the course of 4 weeks, her confusion, edema, and dyspnea regressed, and her mobility improved. During the course of 6 months, her appetite returned, and she gained about 8 lb (not in edema). The activities and spiritual director worked with her to help identify therapeutic and distracting activities for her. The family was pleased with the outcome, and she is stable 2 years later with no hospitalizations. The development of this program was sponsored by a local charitable institution and was a joint project of the nursing home, a local hospice agency, and the Cleveland Clinic. Once running, the program typically had 3 active residents at any time (out of a facility of 100 beds) and required 1 hour-long interdisciplinary meeting twice each month.

Finally, the impact of the rising use of assisted living facilities (ALFs) on health disparities is unclear but concerning. There are now nearly a million elders in ALFs.[28] They are approximately the same age as those who reside in nursing homes, have a high prevalence of cognitive impairment, and are impaired in 2 basic activities of daily living. In the ALF, residents or their families retain responsibility for tending to their health care needs, and as a result, there is much less governmental oversight or data collection. Additionally, the overwhelming majority of ALFs accept private pay only. ALF cost is unaffordable for low- or moderate-income elders, unless they use assets as well as income to pay. The overall impact of the ALFs may be to siphon elders with the highest financial resources (usually whites) away from the nursing homes, leaving a higher proportion of residents (usually nonwhites) who rely on Medicaid facilities for care. If health care in nursing homes that rely heavily on Medicaid reimbursement continues to be bottom tier in terms of structural and performance measures of quality, then health care disparities for minorities will persist or even worsen with the growth of private-pay ALFs.

SUMMARY

Addressing the Healthy People 2010 goal of eliminating health disparities in the nursing home requires addressing facility and payer issues in addition to all the factors that contribute to health disparities in the community. The continued segregation of minority residents in facilities that rely heavily on Medicaid suggests a target for government intervention. Increasing Medicaid reimbursement may help reduce disparities, since there is evidence that Medicaid does not currently cover the basic cost of care. Increasing the coverage of Medicaid in ALFs and community care may stem the growing proportion and further segregation of minority Medicaid recipients in nursing home facilities. Requiring more education in geriatric principles and increased use of geriatric specialists in the nursing home (both physician and mid-level extender) may improve chronic disease care, reduce polypharmacy, and reduce hospital admissions. More disincentives to use PIMs, which may preferentially and adversely affect African Americans and those with Medicaid, may improve care in all facilities. Eliminating nonfinancial promoters of segregation, such as religious restrictions, may help desegregate facilities. When facilities have larger resources from non-Medicaid sources, they can support more staff and services, potentially benefiting all residents in the nursing home regardless of race and ethnicity.

REFERENCES

1. U.S. Department of Health and Human Services. Healthy people 2010: understanding and improving health. 2nd edition. Washington, DC: U.S. Government Printing Office; 2000.
2. National Center for Health Statistics. Health, United States, 2007 with chartbook on trends in the health of Americans. Hyattsville (MD): U.S. Government Printing Office; 2007.
3. Cleeland CS, Gonin R, Baez L, et al. Pain and treatment of pain in minority patients with cancer. The eastern cooperative oncology group minority outpatient pain study. Ann Intern Med 1997;127(9):813–6.
4. Jha AK, Fisher ES, Li Z, et al. Racial trends in the use of major procedures among the elderly. N Engl J Med 2005;353(7):683–91.
5. Brock DB, Foley DJ. Demography and epidemiology of dying in the U.S. with emphasis on deaths of older persons. Hosp J 1998;13(1–2):49–60.
6. Strahan GW. An overview of nursing homes and their current residents: data from the 1995 national nursing home survey. In: Advance Data From Vital and Health Statistics. Hyattsville (MD): National Center for Health Statistics; 1997. p. 1–12.
7. National Nursing Home Survey. Characteristics, staffing, and management (tables 1-10). Bethesda (MD): Center for Disease Control; 2006.
8. Smith DB, Feng Z, Fennell ML, et al. Separate and unequal: racial segregation and disparities in quality across U.S. nursing homes. Health Aff (Millwood) 2007;26(5):1448–58.
9. Seidman B. A briefing chartbook on shortfalls in medicaid funding for nursing home care. American Health Care Association. Available at: https://www.nescsontrak.com/HomePage/files/seidmanstudy0207.pdf. Accessed March 31, 2009.
10. Mor V, Zinn J, Angelelli J, et al. Driven to tiers: socioeconomic and racial disparities in the quality of nursing home care. Milbank Q 2004;82(2):227–56.
11. Lau DT, Kasper JD, Potter DE, et al. Potentially inappropriate medication prescriptions among elderly nursing home residents: their scope and associated resident and facility characteristics. Health Serv Res 2004;39(5):1257–76.
12. Spooner JJ, Lapane KL, Hume AL, et al. Pharmacologic treatment of diabetes in long-term care. J Clin Epidemiol 2001;54(5):525–30.
13. Latif A, Peng X, Messinger-Rapport B. Predictors of anticoagulation prescription in nursing home residents with atrial fibrillation. J Am Med Dir Assoc 2005;6:128–31.
14. National Nursing Home Survey. Employee vaccinations (tables 21–23). Bethesda (MD): Center for Disease Control; 2006.
15. Gruneir A, Miller SC, Feng Z, et al. Relationship between state Medicaid policies, nursing home racial composition, and the risk of hospitalization for black and white residents. Health Serv Res 2008;43(3):869–81.
16. Intrator O, Zinn J, Mor V. Nursing home characteristics and potentially preventable hospitalizations of long-stay residents. J Am Geriatr Soc 2004;52(10):1730–6.
17. Teno JM, Clarridge BR, Casey V, et al. Family perspectives on end-of-life care at the last place of care. JAMA 2004;291(1):88–93.
18. National Nursing Home Survey. Programs and services (tables 11–20). Bethesda (MD): Center for Disease Control; 2006.
19. Messinger-Rapport BJ, Kamel HK. Predictors of do not resuscitate orders in the nursing home. J Am Med Dir Assoc 2005;6(1):18–21.

20. Degenholtz HB, Arnold RA, Meisel A, et al. Persistence of racial disparities in advance care plan documents among nursing home residents. J Am Geriatr Soc 2002;50(2):378–81.
21. Mitchell SL, Teno JM, Roy J, et al. Clinical and organizational factors associated with feeding tube use among nursing home residents with advanced cognitive impairment. JAMA 2003;290(1):73–80.
22. Fairrow AM, McCallum T, Messinger-Rapport B. Preferences of older African Americans for long-term tube feeding at the end of life. Aging Ment Health 2004;8(6):530–4.
23. Fama T, Fox PD. Efforts to improve primary care delivery to nursing home residents. J Am Geriatr Soc 1997;45(5):627–32.
24. Katz PR, Karuza J. The nursing home physician workforce. J Am Med Dir Assoc 2006;7(6):394–7 [discussion: 397–8].
25. Katz PR, Karuza J, Kolassa J, et al. Medical practice with nursing home residents: results from the national physician professional activities census. J Am Geriatr Soc 1997;45(8):911–7.
26. Elon R. Nursing home reform and the governance of medicine: lessons from Maryland. J Am Med Dir Assoc 2002;3(2):73–8.
27. Levenson S. The Maryland regulations: rethinking physician and medical director accountability in nursing homes. J Am Med Dir Assoc 2002;3(2):79–94.
28. Polzer K. Assisted living state regulatory review 2009. National Center for Assisted Living. Available at: http://www.ncal.org/about/state_review.cfm. Accessed March 31, 2009.

Falls in the Nursing Home: A Collaborative Approach

Barbara Messinger-Rapport, MD, PhD, CMD, FACP[a,b,*],
Linda G. Dumas, PhD, RN, ANP-BC[c]

KEYWORDS

- Falls • Delirium • Polypharmacy • Urinary incontinence
- Stroke rehabilitation • Vitamin D

Falls are the most frequently reported adverse event in the nursing home (NH). Consequences can range from minimal to severe. Although we used to think of falls as the inevitable consequence of age and functional decline, we now view falls as the result of potentially modifiable risk factors. Older adults in the NH are heterogeneous. Some are cognitively alert and physically frail. Others are cognitively impaired but physically robust. Most have varying degrees of cognitive and physical impairment. Interventions, then, are heterogeneous as well and tailored to the individual and the facility. Problem solving to reduce fall risk must account for and individualize medical, nursing, and facility factors. For the purposes of this article, the authors, a geriatrician and a gerontological nurse practitioner, offer a case-based, collaborative approach to assessing the falls in 4 residents whom we think you will recognize.

BACKGROUND

About 40% of NH residents fall yearly, and many fall more than once.[1,2] About 35% of falls in NHs occur among patients who cannot walk.[3] Many of the residents in NHs had a history of falls and fall-related injury in the community before admission, often resulting in NH admission. Persons who fall are at risk of future falls. Thus, the prevalence of falls in nursing is *much higher* than it is in the community.

Consequences of falls can be significant even when there is no apparent injury. Among the elderly who are ambulatory following a fall, many develop a fear of falling and decreased willingness to perform functional activities, such as bathing, dressing,

[a] Section of Geriatric Medicine, Cleveland Clinic, Mail Code A91, 9500 Euclid Avenue, Cleveland, OH 44195, USA
[b] Cleveland Clinic Lerner College of Medicine, Case Western Reserve University, Mail Code A91, 9500 Euclid Avenue, Cleveland, OH 44195, USA
[c] College of Nursing and Health Sciences, University of Massachusetts Boston, 100 Morrissey Boulevard, Science Building, Third Floor, Room 300 71, Boston, MA 02125, USA
* Corresponding author. Section of Geriatric Medicine, Cleveland Clinic, Mail Code A91, 9500 Euclid Avenue, Cleveland, OH 44195.
E-mail address: rapporb@ccf.org (B. Messinger-Rapport).

Nurs Clin N Am 44 (2009) 187–195
doi:10.1016/j.cnur.2009.03.001
0029-6465/09/$ – see front matter © 2009 Elsevier Inc. All rights reserved.
nursing.theclinics.com

and walking.[4] Such individuals often become socially isolated.[5] NH residents, because of their frailty, have disproportionate rates of hip fracture and higher mortality rates than their community counterparts.[6] About 10% to 20% of falls in NHs cause serious injuries, and 2% to 6% cause fractures.[6] Facilities are expected to use falls and fall risk (according to the Minimum Data Set [MDS] and any other tools used by the facility) to initiate the Resident Assessment Protocol (RAP). A resident care plan is individualized according to clues that may emerge from the RAP. Prevalence of falls in a facility is a quality indicator and must be reported to federal regulators, who use this information to target facility surveys. Surveyors will look at the MDS, the RAP, and the care plans to see if appropriate attention has been given to fall risk and whether the care plan is individualized to the resident.

Causes of falls in older adults are usually classified into *extrinsic causes* (such as poor lighting, uneven surface, or being pushed) and *intrinsic causes* (dizziness, lower-extremity weakness, gait disorders, and infection). In the community, *predictors* of serious fall injuries include cognitive impairment, 2 or more chronic comorbidities, balance and gait impairments, low BMI, and female gender.[7]

However, in an NH, these factors are endemic. Most of the residents are female, most have multiple comorbidities, and nearly two-thirds of residents take 9 or more medications.[8,9]

Most falls and fall-related injuries in the NH likely result from the intrinsic resident characteristics associated with aging and illness, including multiple medical problems, osteoporosis, urinary incontinence, dementia, anemia, and mobility impairments. Only 10% of NH falls may be attributed solely to environmental hazards, such as inappropriate flooring, poor lighting, and seating areas without grab bars or chair arms.[1] Even when falls are attributed to an *extrinsic problem*, such as an environmental hazard, comorbidities are so prevalent in residents that their *intrinsic characteristics* increase the risk of a fall or fall-related injury.

FALLS IN THE NURSING HOME
Polypharmacy

Polypharmacy, a result of multiple comorbidities, is associated with falls in multiple studies. Drugs from specific classes, including antidepressants, neuroleptic agents, benzodiazepines, anticonvulsants, and class IA antiarrhythmic medications, appear associated with falls fairly consistently.[10] Although hypnotics are classically implicated in falls in older adults, recent evidence suggests that insomnia itself may increase the risk for falls.[11] Moreover, although the older, tricyclic antidepressants are classically associated with falls, newer antidepressants, such as the selective serotonin reuptake inhibitors (SSRIs), are implicated as well.[12]

In a nationally representative sample of NHs, risk factors for fractures included age 85 years and more, admission from the community, agitation, and use of an assistive device.[11] Use of anticonvulsants, antidepressants, opioid analgesics, iron supplements, bisphosphonates, thiazides, and laxatives was associated with fractures. The nurse/certified aide ratio was highly associated with more fractures. The nurse/resident ratio was also associated with more falls.

Potentially inappropriate medications (PIMs) may be implicated in falls when there are psychotropic changes (including delirium) as a result of the medication. A list of PIMs may be found in the "Beers" list in the United States.[13,14] (a periodically updated list of PIMs developed by expert consensus, published by Dr. M.H. Beers) and in the Screening Tool of Older Persons' potentially inappropriate Prescriptions list in Europe.[15] Centers for Medicare and Medicaid Services uses the 1997 Beers list in its new F-Tag 428 during surveys. Reducing the number of medications, particularly those with psychotropic properties, may decrease the risk of falls and fall-related injury.

Case I

Ms. Sadd, 82 years old, has fallen 3 times in the past month. Citalopram was started 6 weeks ago for a major depressive disorder, and since then her mood has improved tremendously. The pharmacist leaves you a note on the chart that antidepressants are associated with falls and fractures and "clinical correlation required." There is no fever, abdominal pain, dysuria, or change in her urinary habits. You check a urinalysis and find it positive, with more than 100,000 Escherichia coli present.

Your approach

You have uncovered asymptomatic bacteriuria in your resident, and although it will likely resolve temporarily with antibiotic treatment, her fall risk will not be altered. You reduce the dose of citalopram from 20 mg to 10 mg. She falls once the next day, and then has no falls during the next month. You reassess her medications and notice that she is not receiving any supplements of calcium or vitamin D.

Vitamin D and Falls in the Nursing Home

Vitamin D insufficiency is common in fractures of women in long-term care (LTC), and more than half the women in LTC are deficient in vitamin D.[16,17] Newer recommendations for vitamin D intake for at risk elders is 1000 U daily.[18] LTC facilities typically supply less than 200 U of vitamin D in a typical diet.[19] Supplementation in both men and women of vitamin D 800 U can decrease the risk of falls.[20] Calcium supplementation is needed as well. Because of the controversy linking high intake of calcium to increased cardiovascular events in older adults,[21] the typical NH diet should be supplemented up to 1,000 mg daily. Keep in mind that if a resident is receiving supplements such as Ensure or Boost, or tube feeding, these products are already heavily supplemented with calcium (although not with much vitamin D), so additional calcium may not be needed.

Treatments for osteoporosis will not alter the fall risk in mobile residents but may reduce the risk of fall-related injuries. Bisphosphonates reduce the risk of hip fractures by approximately 50% in community women with low bone density[22] and decrease the risk of vertebral fracture in women 80 years and older by about 80%.[23] In those residents unable to swallow pills safely, a yearly infusion of zoledronic acid is effective in reducing the risk of fracture.[24] Teriparatide reduces the risk of vertebral and nonvertebral fractures in postmenopausal women but is expensive and requires a daily injection.[25] Duration of use is limited by the Food and Drug Administration to 2 years. Hip protectors were shown in one study by Kannus and colleagues[26] to reduce the risk of hip fractures in a clustered NH study, but their results have not been replicated.[27] There are no studies for calcium, bisphosphonates, or teriparatide in bed-bound NH residents, and there may be risks in their use.[28]

Continuation of Case

You start Ms. Sadd on 1000 U daily of vitamin D3 (cholecalciferol). She is lactose intolerant, so you administer 2 500-mg Tums each evening. A bone-density test reveals osteopenia but not osteoporosis. You discuss hip protectors with the family and decide not to use them right now. Each pair costs about $100, is not reimbursable by insurance, and is not definitively shown to reduce the risk of fracture.

Urinary Incontinence

Urinary incontinence, a risk factor for falls and fractures, is present in more than 50% of NH residents.[29] Unfortunately, even medications that are not PIMs may increase urinary incontinence. Such medications include the cholinesterase inhibitors such as donepezil, galantamine, and rivastigmine. A growing body of literature links the SSRI class of antidepressants, as well as mirtazapine and venlafaxine, to urinary incontinence.[30,31] Additionally, since edema is redistributed at night, resulting in increased nocturnal urination and incontinence, medications that increase edema (such as amlodipine or Felodipine) may increase the risk of incontinence. Finally, antimuscarinic medications, such as Detrol, used to treat urinary urge incontinence, are potentially inappropriate in elders with dementia[15] and may increase the risk of confusion and falls.

Case II

Ms. Night is a lovely 88-year-old woman with mild dementia, hypertension, and edema, taking amlodipine 10 mg and Donepezil 10 mg daily. She has nocturia up to 10 times per night and wakes up wet each morning. She fell rushing to the toilet. The family asks for a sleeping pill and one of the new medications they read about for overactive bladder.

Your approach

You ask restorative nursing to monitor her urination pattern and confirm that she really is urinating 10 times between 9:00 PM and 6:00 AM. Prescribing a sleeping pill may increase the risk of confusion and thus falls at night. The antimuscarinic medications for the overactive bladder are relatively contraindicated in dementia. You lower the dose of Donepezil to 5 mg. You decrease the dose of amlodipine to 5 mg and add a low dose of hydrochlorothiazide (12.5 mg) in the morning. After 2 weeks, her edema is minimal, and her blood pressure is controlled. Restorative nursing evaluates her voiding pattern and finds that she now awakens only 3 to 4 times each evening and stays dry.

Additional interventions include placing a stable commode next to her bed (or moving her bed nearer to the bathroom at night); making sure that there is a nightlight in the room; and offering a course of physical therapy to improve mobility. The family is happy with the outcome of these interventions. There are vitamin D receptors in the urogenital system, so you also add the vitamin D 1,000 supplement and Tums to provide calcium in addition to decreasing the fall risk and risk of fall-related injury.

Delirium

Delirium is a common problem in the NH and is associated with falls. Delirium may be a result of an inappropriate medication or of an underlying condition, such as an infection. An unexplained fall in a resident without a history of falls may actually be a "sentinel" fall, sentinel in the sense that there is a new underlying condition hitherto undetected by the facility staff. Elderly residents may in fact have a nonspecific presentation of an illness, so pneumonia, for example, may not actually present with a fever and cough, but with confusion, loss of continence, and a fall. All facilities employ an assessment protocol following a resident's fall. In one clinical trial, a resident assessment within 7 days following a fall did not reduce the risk of future falls but did reduce the risk of subsequent hospitalization and of the number of hospital days.[3] Once a fall triggers the cascade of extra nursing attention, the delirium is uncovered, and the underlying condition (such as infection) may be treated promptly.

Case III

Mr. Strong is a 90-year-old man who is usually continent, ambulatory, and had not fallen during the 2 years he had been at the facility. The daughter reported that he was a bit sleepy the previous week and smelled strongly of urine. The next day he fell in the hallway. He appeared to be without injury and had no complaints. He was able to ambulate immediately after the fall.

Your approach

Your facility has a protocol that is followed after every fall. It involves a nursing assessment, vital signs immediately, then during every shift for 3 days, and then daily to complete a 7-day period. The case of each resident who has fallen is discussed in the weekly falls committee for the next month to identify interventions and to monitor for improvement.

Vital signs were 97.5 F temperature, 102 beats per minute pulse, 20 respirations per minute, and 122/80 mm Hg blood pressure. The nursing assessment revealed crackles at the bases of both lung fields and new inattentiveness. He is polite but disinterested, sits by the window, and does not interact with staff. Vital signs and a nursing assessment were checked each shift as per protocol. The next recorded temperature shows 100.5, and he is now complaining of a dry cough. You order a chest x-ray and find pneumonia. With oral antibiotics and having the aides encourage fluids, he does well. This week he is stronger, ambulating more confidently, and is continent again. He returned to his attentive, interactive, sociable self. There were no more falls.

With Mr. Strong, close nursing attention and the interdisciplinary fall evaluation demonstrated that this fall was actually a "sentinel fall" preceding the diagnosis of an infection. He presented with a hypoactive delirium and new incontinence. This fall exemplifies the nonspecific presentation of illness arising in elderly residents. LTC facilities employ an assessment protocol following a resident's fall. In one clinical trial, a resident assessment within 7 days following a fall did not reduce the risk of future falls but did reduce the risk of subsequent hospitalization and of the number of hospital days.[3] Had his fall not initiated the cascade of extra nursing attention, his pneumonia would have progressed to dehydration and hypoxia, and he would have required admission. With the intervention, his pneumonia was treated and his delirium resolved.

COMPREHENSIVE APPROACH TO THE FALL DURING REHABILITATION

Case IV

Mr. Stroker is in our rehabilitation section of the facility recovering from a stroke. He has a dense left hemiparesis and needs full assistance for all activities of daily living. Because of dysphagia, he had a percutaneous endoscopic gastrostomy (PEG) tube placed before hospital discharge, and it is running continuously at 75 cc/h. He has been restless while sitting, often shifting position. He is able to speak but has not offered an explanation to the nurses about his need to change position. He has been ambulating with assistance in therapy, but yesterday, while in the lobby in his wheelchair, he tried to rise without assistance. He became tangled up in his tube-feeding apparatus and fell forward, pulling the wheelchair and the entire feeding apparatus on top of him. Because of severe wrist and left-hip pain, 911 was summoned, and he spent 2 days in the hospital. Fortunately, other than contusions and pain, he was not seriously injured. His rehabilitation process, however, slowed down tremendously.

After a patient's fall, the nurse is legally required to notify the medical director or nurse practitioner on call, as well as the family. Nursing intervention after a fall should include an immediate, problem-focused assessment to determine if it was witnessed, whether the resident is injured, if he hit his head, the location of pain, and a passive range of motion to assess for fracture or dislocation. Head trauma and hip fracture are serious consequences of falls.[6] Either can lead to long-term cognitive impairment and functional decline. Many facilities will have protocols for emergency evaluation for each head injury or unwitnessed fall that may be a head injury to identify an intracranial hemorrhage.

Assessment and intervention after a fall require a good knowledge of health assessment, the ability to do a problem-focused assessment, and how to ask questions about the history of the event. It is important that nurses know the reasons why NHs are sites for significantly higher fall rates and serious sequelae to the fall event.

In the case of Mr. Stroker, questions should be asked about his risk factors for a fall, which risk factors can be modified, and which are nonmodifiable. Nonmodifiable risk factors could be some of the intrinsic conditions, such as advanced age and cognitive impairment gait; modifiable risk factors are many of the extrinsic risk factors and some of the intrinsic ones, such as infection, delirium, number of medications, adverse drug effect, vitamin or mineral deficiency, and mobility. What are the comorbidities and which are the causes of the fall? This patient had been seriously ill poststroke; his fall left him with more comorbidities, such as bruises, pain, and potentially impaired rehabilitation, if he develops significant fear of falling.

The first nursing consideration postfall relates to the PEG apparatus and tubing. His tube feeding schedule could be changed from continuous to intermittent with the TF off when he is up in his wheelchair. This change limits the times during the day when he could become entangled in the apparatus, causing a fall or injury. This is an example where the nurses, therapists, and other personnel such as dietary consultants can be creative when individualizing resident treatment.

Stroke patients are often depressed during recovery, especially in early recovery when goals seem insurmountable. As a result, many eat poorly. A second nursing intervention is optimizing his nutrition. Adequate nutrition is a critical factor for his recovery along with the physical, occupational, and speech therapy condition following a stroke. There are several relevant nursing and dietary staff teaching points about his PEG feedings. His feeding is Jevity 1500 mL/24 h. This quantity of tube feeding provides 460 IU vitamin D3 and 1370 mg calcium daily, which is insufficient in vitamin D. Further calcium supplementation may increase the risk of kidney stones, but he needs another 600 U daily of vitamin D to reduce his falls and fracture risk. Collaboration with the dietary consultants is important to optimize his nutritional needs.

Osteoporosis issues should also be addressed. Stroke patients tend to develop osteoporosis on the weaker side. If tolerated, consideration should be given to a bisphosphonate once ambulatory. He may benefit from an intravenous bisphosphonate since he has dysphagia.

Another nursing intervention for Mr. Stroker is to identify why he is agitated and trying to rise. Does he need more physical activity? Is there a urination issue such as dysuria, frequency, or retention? Is he experiencing discomfort and irritation from painful areas associated with incontinence of urine and stool? Is he in pain from arthritis? The restlessness and agitation that occur with chronic illness, incontinence, dementia, and chronic pain require best-practice nursing assessment and interventions.

In the case of Mr. Stroker, he has returned from the hospital with injuries that are not serious but painful. Pain management should begin as soon as he returns to the NH.

Consider Tylenol for mild chronic pain; for moderate to severe pain due to his fall to the floor, cautious use of tramadol, hydrocodone, or oxycodone would be appropriate. Since he may have pain but not ask for any medications, consider scheduling 1 gm of Tylenol 3 times daily for 3 to 5 days following a significant fall. An informal or formal assessment of pain should occur with each patient encounter to determine if a pain medication is needed. Pain medications require consistent attention to side effects and drug interactions.

NURSING INTERVENTIONS TO PREVENT FALLS—ASSESSING THE FACILITY'S CULTURE
Primary, Secondary, and Tertiary Prevention

An important question is how do we change the culture of NHs to improve safety and bring best practice to everyday life in the facility?[6] One of the best ways is through nursing and nurse assistant education on a regular basis. The medical director, director of nursing, and nurse educator should implement an ongoing series of patient-focused seminars on causes, consequences, and prevention of falls in the NH. Quality indicators should be identified and complied with. Preventive strategies should be behavior based, creative, and individualized to the resident. Physical and occupational therapy may prevent falls as well.

Other preventive nursing interventions are based on a thorough and ongoing assessment of the patient. *Extrinsic* or environmental modifications are easiest to introduce quickly. Lowered beds, side rails at the head of the bed, and floor mats next to the bed in case of a fall are routine nurse interventions when a patient at risk comes to the unit. Rooms and halls should be brightly lit.

Regular vision testing and podiatry are required by law for NHs. Poor vision has been shown to be a cause of falls.[32] Painful feet are another fall risk, and the risk may be reduced with properly fitting shoes. Podiatrists routinely visit NH residents every 3 months.

Alarm sensors for chair, bed, and even toilet may help alert staff that a resident needs immediate attention. Restraints should be avoided since they may not decrease the risk of falls and injuries. A geri chair may be used for those with specific repositioning needs but may be considered a restraint, thus used only judiciously.

It is emphasized that best practices require excellent assessment skills, mentoring, and a creative application of knowledge to individual patients. The culture of the NHs will not change without educated nurses, educated certified nursing assistants, and administrators who are involved with care on the units.[6]

An etiology of falls that was not specifically discussed here is mental illness. Polypharmacy and use of inappropriate drugs for frail older adults with multiple comorbidities have been discussed. These are common etiologies of falls in patients with mental illness, dementia, psychosis, or behavioral issues. Geriatric nurse clinicians and psychiatrists partner with NHs and have become a presence and another resource for staff. Schizophrenia and dementia are intrinsic and significant risk factors for falls.[33]

SUMMARY

In this article, falls were discussed with a team approach by a geriatrician and a geriatric nurse practitioner. Improving the quality of lives in NHs, maximizing safety, managing pain, and educating NH nurses and staff about fall safety and prevention are the nursing objectives for the residents of LTC. Collaborative approaches that are individualized and "creative" make sense, as the body of evidence-based interventions in the NH grows.[34]

Most are evidence based; a few just make good sense. Nurses in LTC can conduct small clinical research studies to build on the body of evidence-based practice in falls. LTC facilities are communities; they are homes. Partnerships between physicians and nurse providers are optimal with their shared, but different, expertise. We, as nurses and physicians, share a responsibility for the protection of NH residents, most of whom are vulnerable, compromised, and cannot speak for themselves.

REFERENCES

1. Nurmi I, Luthje P. Incidence and costs of falls and fall injuries among elderly in institutional care. Scand J Prim Health Care 2002;20(2):118–22.
2. Luukinen H, Koski K, Honkanen R, et al. Incidence of injury-causing falls among older adults by place of residence: a population-based study. J Am Geriatr Soc 1995;43(8):871–6.
3. Rubenstein LZ, Robbins AS, Josephson KR, et al. The value of assessing falls in an elderly population. A randomized clinical trial. Ann Intern Med 1990;113(4): 308–16.
4. Arfken CL, Lach HW, Birge SJ, et al. The prevalence and correlates of fear of falling in elderly persons living in the community. Am J Public Health 1994; 84(4):565–70.
5. Cooper C, Campion G, Melton L III. Hip fractures in the elderly: a world-wide projection. Osteoporos Int 1992;2:285–92.
6. Magaziner J, Miller R, Resnick B. Intervening to prevent falls and fractures in nursing homes: are we putting the cart before the horse? J Am Geriatr Soc 2007;55(3):464–6. Available at: www.medscape.com. Accessed February 15, 2009.
7. Tinetti M, Doucette J, Claus E, et al. Risk factors for serious injury during falls by older persons in the community. J Am Geriatr Soc 1995;43(11):1214–21.
8. Centers for disease Control and Prevention. Injury center, falls in nursing homes. Washington, DC: Centers for Disease Control and Prevention; 2009. Accessed February 15, 2009.
9. Rubenstein LZ. Preventing falls in the nursing home. JAMA 1997;278(7):595–6.
10. Tinetti ME. Clinical practice. Preventing falls in elderly persons. N Engl J Med 2003;348(1):42–9.
11. Spector W, Shaffer T, Potter DE, et al. Risk factors associated with the occurrence of fractures in U.S. nursing homes: resident and facility characteristics and prescription medications. J Am Geriatr Soc 2007;55(3):327–33.
12. Ensrud KE, Blackwell TL, Mangione CM, et al. Central nervous system-active medications and risk for falls in older women. J Am Geriatr Soc 2002;50(10): 1629–37.
13. Beers MH. Explicit criteria for determining potentially inappropriate medication use by the elderly. An update. Arch Intern Med 1997;157(14):1531–6.
14. Fick DM, Cooper JW, Wade WE, et al. Updating the beers criteria for potentially inappropriate medication use in older adults: Results of a US consensus panel of experts. Arch Intern Med 2003;163(22):2716–24.
15. Gallagher P, O'Mahony D. STOPP (screening tool of older persons' potentially inappropriate prescriptions): application to acutely ill elderly patients and comparison with beers' criteria. Age Ageing 2008;37(6):673–9.
16. Elliott ME, Binkley NC, Carnes M, et al. Fracture risks for women in long-term care: High prevalence of calcaneal osteoporosis and hypovitaminosis d. Pharmacotherapy 2003;23(6):702–10.

17. Pieper CF, Colon-Emetic C, Caminis J, et al. Distribution and correlates of serum 25-hydroxyvitamin d levels in a sample of patients with hip fracture. Am J Geriatr Pharmacother 2007;5(4):335–40.
18. U.S. Department of Health and Human Services. U.S. Department of Agriculture. Dietary guidelines for Americans. 6th edition. Washington, DC: U.S. Government Printing Office; 2005.
19. Johnson RM, Smiciklas-Wright H, Soucy IM, et al. Nutrient intake of nursing-home residents receiving pureed foods or a regular diet. J Am Geriatr Soc 1995;43(4):344–8.
20. Broe KE, Chen TC, Weinberg J, et al. A higher dose of vitamin d reduces the risk of falls in nursing home residents: a randomized, multiple-dose study. J Am Geriatr Soc 2007;55(2):234–9.
21. Bolland MJ, Barber PA, Doughty RN, et al. Vascular events in healthy older women receiving calcium supplementation: randomised controlled trial. BMJ 2008;336(7638):262–6.
22. Black D, Cumings S, Karpf D, et al. Randomised trial of effect of alendronate on risk of fracture in women with existing vertebral fractures. Fracture intervention trial research group. Lancet 1996;348(9041):1535–41.
23. Boonen S, McClung MR, Eastell R, et al. Safety and efficacy of risedronate in reducing fracture risk in osteoporotic women aged 80 and older: implications for the use of antiresorptive agents in the old and oldest old. J Am Geriatr Soc 2004;52(11):1832–9.
24. Black DM, Delmas PD, Eastell R, et al. Once-yearly zoledronic acid for treatment of postmenopausal osteoporosis. N Engl J Med 2007;356(18):1809–22.
25. Neer RM, Arnaud CD, Zanchetta JR, et al. Effect of parathyroid hormone (1-34) on fractures and bone mineral density in postmenopausal women with osteoporosis. N Engl J Med 2001;344(19):1434–41.
26. Kannus P, Parkkari J, Niemi S, et al. Prevention of hip fracture in elderly people with use of a hip protector. N Engl J Med 2000;343(21):1506–13.
27. Kiel DP, Magaziner J, Zimmerman S, et al. Efficacy of a hip protector to prevent hip fracture in nursing home residents: the hip pro randomized controlled trial. JAMA 2007;298(4):413–22.
28. Kamel HK. Update on osteoporosis management in long-term care: focus on bisphosphonates. J Am Med Dir Assoc 2007;8(7):434–40.
29. Sgadari A, Topinkova E, Bjornson J, et al. Urinary incontinence in nursing home residents: a cross-national comparison. Age Ageing 1997;26(Suppl 2):49–54.
30. Cavanaugh GL, Martin RE, Stenson MA, et al. Venlafaxine and urinary incontinence: possible association. Ann Pharmacother 1997;31(3):372.
31. Votolato NA, Stern S, Caputo RM. Serotonergic antidepressants and urinary incontinence. Int Urogynecol J Pelvic Floor Dysfunct 2000;11(6):386–8.
32. Cummings R, Ivers R, Clemson L, et al. Improving vision to prevent falls in frail older people. A randomized trial. J Am Geriatr Soc 2007;55(2):175–81.
33. Rayner. A. Managing psychotic symptoms in the older patient geriatrics and aging 2007;10(4):241–5.
34. Messinger-Rapport BJ. Evidence-based medicine: is it relevant to long-term care? J Am Med Dir Assoc 2004;5(5):328–32.

Pain Management in the Nursing Home

Linda G. Dumas, PhD, RN, ANP-BC[a],*, Murali Ramadurai, MD, CMD[b]

KEYWORDS

- Nursing home • Acute • Chronic • End of life
- Transitional care • Symptom burden • Anxiety

The articles on hospice and end-of-life care in this issue reflect a philosophy and ways of looking at illness, life, and death—concepts that are unfamiliar to many long-term care (LTC) providers. This article is specifically about pain management and some of the best practices to address the problem of pain in nursing home patients who have a serious illness and multiple comorbid conditions. Pain management is at the core of the work of nurse practitioners and physicians. Best practices include a sound knowledge of medications, their effectiveness, their interactions, and how they are used in the very sick, the old, and the most compromised adults; the importance of a knowledge of renal function and its relationship to pain medications cannot be overstated. The management of pain at the end of life is often reflective of palliative care and hospice philosophy. Pain management for patients in short-term care, pain management for LTC patients with chronic illness and multiple comorbidities, and pain management at the end of life have different goals.

Management of the emotional distress that accompanies chronic or acute pain is of foremost concern. Providers need to be experts in assessing psychosocial and physical issues. Many have expertise; few are really comfortable in the pain management role.

Topics discussed in this article include the following: first, general pain management in a nursing home for a LTC resident who has chronic pain; second, the relief of symptoms and suffering in a patient who is on palliative care and hospice; and third, the pain management of a postoperative patient with acute pain for a short transitional period (post–acute illness or surgery). All are connected by goals related to relief of symptom burden, suffering, and the diffuse anxiety that often accompanies both. The context of illness and pain are unique to each individual. The same medication, such as morphine, may be used in very different ways.

[a] Department of Nursing, University of Massachusetts Boston, College of Nursing and Health Sciences, 100 Morrissey Boulevard, Boston, MA 02125, USA
[b] American Board of Internal Medicine, American Board of Hospice and Palliative Medicine, Senior Health Care Associates, Inc., 83 Littlefield Road, Newton, MA 02459, USA
* Corresponding author.
E-mail address: linda.dumas@umb.edu (L.G. Dumas).

Nurs Clin N Am 44 (2009) 197–208
doi:10.1016/j.cnur.2009.04.001
0029-6465/09/$ – see front matter © 2009 Elsevier Inc. All rights reserved.
nursing.theclinics.com

Two aspects of pain management are stressed in this article: an introduction to common medications in pain management for acute and chronic pain and end-of-life contexts. The fact that any pain management is ideally an outcome of conversations between staff nurses, nurse practitioners, and physicians is emphasized. It is also an outcome of evidence-based practice. Pain management cannot and should not be separated from the psychosocial distress that emerges from the presence of pain in one's life. Worry, anxiety, and fear loom large as one suffers more refractory pain. Some of the moral issues that arise when caring for patients with pain are also examined. People with pain are more vulnerable because of how they feel and because, as patients, they are dependent on providers. They are frightened and ill.

Nurses and physicians who become patients have life-altering experiences as the balance shifts from being providers in control to becoming patients. The voice of Graboys,[1] a renowned cardiologist and now a patient with Parkinson disease and Lewy body dementia, speaks for many providers who spent their lives taking care of others. He writes: "Holding on. Much of my life today and every day is about holding on to what I've got, or more precisely is holding on to what I have left."[1] "It is my hope that others who suffer from serious disease, especially those struggling with disease that steals control of mind or body... will find some comfort—that I may be able to articulate, and therefore, validate, what they feel and experience but may not be able to express."[1] There but for fortune—as Sontag[2] so eloquently wrote: "So much of pain management for the chronically ill is learning ourselves 'to walk the walk' with each patient. We cannot separate the experience of *illness* from the management of the pain that emanates from the *disease.*"

Ferrell, a nurse and expert on pain management, writes about a "moral crisis of untreated pain."[3] She writes of a "serious undertreatment of pain" that continues despite major advances in medicine.[3] She applies a feminist ethic to the problem of untreated pain and focuses on pain as an existential experience for those who suffer from it. She stresses the role of nursing and "what it means to be a nurse committed to the relief of pain."[3]

An overview of selected literature on pain management in nursing homes is discussed in the next section. One case is presented here with comments from the view of an adult nurse practitioner in geriatrics (L.G.D.) and from the perspective of a physician and expert in palliative care and hospice medicine (M.R.). An important part of what the authors say is showing, by example, the necessity of a strong collaboration and mutual trust between the advanced practice nurse and the physician.

AN OVERVIEW OF SELECTED LITERATURE

The literature in nursing and medicine has become a forum for philosophic discussions of palliative care; palliative care is emerging as an important choice for families of LTC residents with advanced dementias and chronic disease. There is new interest in palliative care programs for nursing home residents as families want comfort care and relief from suffering over time. The distinctions between the presence of hospice in nursing homes and the practice of palliative care sometimes blur. It is projected that 43% of people 65 years and older in 1990 will reside in a nursing home at least once before they die.[4] Of this group, 55% will reside at least 1 year in the nursing home and 21% will reside 21 years or more. The average annual cost for nursing home care will be approximately $125,000. Kane and Kane[4] as well as Kemper and Murtaugh[5] call for imaginative, alternative approaches to provide a new kind of housing that reflects a community rather than an institution. They call it the "greening of the nursing home." Much remains for discussion about who will occupy these "hotel-like" nursing home alternatives. Kane and Kane's work is cutting-edge, and they are opening doors to new dimensions of LTC. No matter where older adults choose to live, they will grow older and sicker and need more services as years pass by.

Alternative settings will bring new options to older adults who are in good health,but nursing homes will still be needed. Nursing home occupancy rates will rise as the demographics of aging peak at about 70 million over 65 in the year 2050.[6] As more advanced practice nurses become nursing home providers, there is an opportunity for collaborative and integrated care of residents. Managing pain, working with families of residents, and bringing up the difficult topics around advanced directives for care are all critical elements of nursing care.

There are many types of pain: acute pain and chronic pain, with nociceptive or proprioceptive distinctions.[7] In the nursing home, where chronic illness predominates, there are frequent episodes of acute illness, such as urinary tract infections, pneumonia, dehydration, or renal failure. Residents become hospitalized patients and return to the nursing home after inpatient treatment and resolution of the acute problem. A chronic illness is usually long and unrelenting, characterized by exacerbation and remission. Palliative-care patients do not have to be in a critical condition, to be on comfort care. Palliative care is well described by Kenen[8] as easing the symptoms of the sick in multiple settings. The nursing home is just one of the settings.

"The idea is to give patients what they need, when they need it, no matter what their ultimate prognosis."[8] Ideally palliative care should start early and continue for a long time.

Illness trajectories and pain trajectories are unpredictable and unique to each patient.[9] A white paper from the American Association of Retired Persons (AARP) Policy Institute reported that the symptoms, needs, and illness trajectories of dying people are insufficiently recognized by professional caregivers. Opportunities for discussions about palliative care and advanced planning are missed.[9] End-of-life care in nursing homes is becoming more common as partnerships are formed between the LTC facility and a hospice.[9] This facilitates care as residents are allowed to die "at home." "Home" represents safety and familiarity. Nursing homes are homes and communities to many of the men and women who live there. The use of well-trained hospice nurses who share responsibility for the patient's pain management and quality of life is greater in 2009. Decisions about chronic pain, end-of-life care, quality of life, and thoughtful, evidence-based use of medications at end of life are all good decisions. Best-practice end-of-life care includes pain management, and it may include use of intravenous fluids, hydration, and antibiotics, among other choices. These are choices to be made by the resident and his or her family. Research includes the use of opioids, not only at end of life but to try to control chronic pain earlier in life. Transdermal fentanyl is a well-tolerated and increasingly accepted treatment for patients who require strong opioids for nonmalignant conditions.

Libretto discusses cases where chronic, unremitting pain is part of life for many people who are not at the end of life.[10] Rheumatoid arthritis, osteoarthritis, spinal stenosis, fractures, and osteoporosis are examples of non–cancer-related chronic pain.[10] "Chronic pain ranges from 45% to 80% among nursing home residents and is found in 75% of people with advanced cancer. The annual cost of treating chronic pain is estimated to be at 1 billion dollars."[11]

Glajchen further speaks about barriers to treatment related to an overreliance on the rules and constraints that the health care system puts on physicians and advanced practice nurses. Fear of regulatory scrutiny is high on this list. Other provider barriers include level of knowledge about pain management, pain assessment, pain history, and cultural constraints.[11] A knowledge of the pharmacology of opioids and the guidelines for staff nurses, nurse practitioners, and physicians is an imperative.

What are the medications that benefit patients with dementia, dyspnea, failure to thrive, arthritic pain, cancer pain, and anxiety? How do we assess the needs of residents with advanced dementias, and related cognitive deficits? How do we assess the pain of residents who are unable to speak and answer questions? How do we assess emotional pain, depression, and other forms of suffering? Providers should be current on pain management and best practices around prescribing.[12] There is a collaboration between providers and families when decisions are made about the hospitalization of nursing home residents with advanced dementia. The do-not-hospitalize (DNH) directive supports "in place" treatments. Keeping residents in their "homes" as they go to hospice sustains community for resident and family. Decisions such as do-not-resuscitate (DNR), DNH should be directing our management of symptom burden and pain. Researchers, in a nationwide study, examined the prevalence of DNH orders in 91,000 nursing home residents who were 65 years or older and who had advanced dementia. Prevalence ranged from I% in Oklahoma to 26% in Rhode Island.[13] Subsequent multivariate analyses showed that DNH was less likely to be used for minority residents and in corporate-based nursing facilities that were chains, which had lower staffing, including advanced practice nurses or physician assistants. It would be interesting to include the presence or absence of evidence-based pain management guidelines in the multivariate analyses in these facilities.

More providers and families today support a palliative management of acute illness, which is reflective of care in the nursing home rather than transfer to hospital.[13] The study showed that DNH orders vary by region and are *uncommon* among nursing home residents with advanced dementia. The findings suggest that the DNH order and the race of the patient require closer examination. Related interventions include a stronger nurse practitioner presence in homes and a facilitation of family discussions about this option.

Secondly, care discussion about code status is not discussed soon enough. Nursing homes require a code status on admission, but often, it is too late for the patient or resident to make that choice. Research databases for hospitals across the United States reflected poor documentation and a dearth of conversations between physicians and families. Conversations need to occur earlier, before hospitalization or nursing home placement. Casarett's research indicates that more than 25% of Americans die in nursing homes.[14] His work reflects that information about hospice care to families is not enough and that family-patient preferences need to be discussed early on with the physician. Outcomes suggested that given the opportunity, residents would benefit from hospice care. Providers and nursing home staff need to raise the issue to families in the early days of placement.[14]

Concluding this overview of issues relating to management of pain in LTC residents are some general comments about therapeutic outcomes of pain management in the nursing home. Residents have multiple physical and emotional issues that need to be addressed. Adequate pain control is at the top of the list of interventions for the resident. The nursing home population presents with multiple challenges to the most skilled of nurses and physicians: residents are sick, they cannot always speak for themselves, and pain assumes a major portion of symptom burden yet is often undertreated. Most of this review focuses on making the point that efficacy of pain management cannot be optimized without education of bedside and advanced practice providers. New knowledge should help to increase the comfort zone with regard to talking with families, significant others, *and* residents, if possible, about advanced directives, particularly those relating to palliative care. Criteria for palliative care are often nonspecific and based on complex comorbid conditions. Hutt and colleagues point out that structural variables, such as staffing patterns in nursing homes, high staff turnover rates, low physician presence in homes, organizational culture, and low nursing salaries are a few of the organizational barriers.[15] The challenges presented by residents are equally compelling, and multiple medical, social, and psychological issues require strong assessment skills, a knowledge of pharmacology, and an understanding by the staff that nursing home residents have very different sets of problems from their counterparts in the community. The rising number of residents with Alzheimer disease and rising numbers of the oldest old are changing the face of the nursing home.

LTC residents are sick, dependent, and very frail. Their quality of life should be maximized, and comfort is integral to quality. Choices around pain and comfort involve families and providers because many of the residents are unable to speak for themselves. This is an important point. Nurses need excellent assessment skills and must take the time to listen and learn from the residents. Residents and families can be teachers to us. Physicians and nurse practitioners must be knowledgeable about the medications and treatments they prescribe. Decisions should be based on evidence and empathy for the residents and their families. Ferrell writes of caregiver burden and sees pain as a "family experience."[3]

In the next 2 sections, the different roles and professional perspectives of the nurse practitioner and the physician are explored as they collaborate to bring comfort and security to the sick in LTC.

A NURSE PRACTITIONER SPEAKS: ASSESSING THE RESIDENT IN PAIN

…Since I was a child I thought that being sick or injured was the worst thing that could happen to a person…. I came to believe that unless you were reasonably healthy and free of pain, much of the rest of the world would be closed off—and that healing the sick was the most important thing anyone could do.[16]

Angell goes on to say:

Almost all of us will be seriously ill at some point, no matter how much we try to avert it. At that time what we will desperately want is compassionate and highly skilled medical care—doctors and nurses…the essence of a decent healthcare system is still caring for the sick.[16]

I teach in a university college of nursing, and at the beginning of each semester I read Angell's editorial to my students. In health care, we focus so much on personal responsibility, choices, health promotion, and disease prevention, that we tend to overlook why we chose the profession of nursing or medicine. I ask my students to remember that their work is to *heal the sick*, and to care with compassion for as long as it takes, to bring comfort to those who cannot be healed.

The best practices in nursing are based on an integration of clinical expertise and compassion. Like physicians, we are taught the art of the health history and the skills to be good listeners.

When we care for people who are ill and in pain, the process begins with the history and the *patient's story.*

This section is dedicated to the nurses who work in hospitals, nursing homes, or related LTC settings. Many residents present in the nursing home with an acute medical problem. I'm going to use the word *patient* from here on as we are talking about seriously ill nursing home residents. Dr. Ramadurai speaks next about the dosing of opioids, the use of opioids, and the importance of understanding *and* accepting the fact that patients in pain need to have their pain relieved. In the nursing home setting, *it should be a given that when the patient says he or she has pain, the patient needs medication for pain relief.* This does not preclude alternative modalities, but such modalities are optional and are choices of the nurse, the patient, or the family. They may also be recommendations by the physician or nurse practitioner provider. Sometimes none of these happen.

Nurses are first-line connections to the patient and family. It is a privilege based on trust; patients do not know us but trust us with the most intimate details of their lives. Medicine and nursing share this distinction.

No article on pain would be complete without an acknowledgment of the nurse who began it all—Dr. Margo McCaffrey. Ferrell calls her "the godmother" of nursing care of patients in pain.[3] McCaffrey's definition is "*pain is what the person says it is and exists whenever he or she says it does.*"[17] Her work has been paradigmatic in the fields of pain management and nursing. The nursing profession continues to be grateful to her for what she brought to nursing and to our patients.

When the patient says, " I have pain," the assessment for intervention begins. Pain is a common reason for phone calls to the service when I triage for nursing homes; many phone calls from the nurses are similar to the following:

The patient is s/p shoulder fracture and needs more pain medication. Vicodin is not helping the pain. The patient requests another pain medication.

The patient's lower extremity is swollen, red, and hot; the scheduled Tylenol is not touching the patient's pain.

The patient just fell out of bed. She is status post hip fracture and fell again on her hip. She is complaining of pain.

The patient with dementia is restless and agitated. He is grimacing, appears uncomfortable and cries. Tylenol is all he has for pain.

The patient is moaning when he is turned and dressings are changed, but when is not moved he is fine. He has prn medication.

The patient is on prn pain medication. He hasn't had it in 2 days. He has not asked for it.

She needs pain medication but she is allergic to Percocet, oxycontin, oxyco-done, and hydrocodone.

And for the dying:

We have hospice recommendations for a change in Roxanol dose. We want to increase to 15 mg sublingually every 2 hours and 8 mg sublingually every hour as needed. The Ativan is increased to 0.5 mg every 2 hours scheduled.

The patient needs scheduled dosing. She is on 15 mg Roxanol every 4 hours when needed. She can no longer tell us what she needs.

The patient is actively dying. We need to increase the morphine (Roxanol) to 20 mg every hour as needed.

The patient was just admitted from the hospital to nursing home after a stroke. He is aphasic but appears to be uncomfortable. He is pointing to the paralyzed arm and hand. He is crying.

The nursing process is a reliable and valid assessment tool that should be used throughout a nurse's career. It is a method; it is an excellent and easy way to organize data. When I get calls like the above, I make an assumption that the nurse has done a competent assessment of the patient's status, has looked at the chart and the medication record (MAR), and has spoken with the patient, family member, or nursing assistant. I have to make an assumption because I am on the phone and not in the unit. I don't see the patient when I am on call. At least 50% of the calls I get relate to pain medication.

The nursing process method includes assessment, diagnosis, planning, implementation, and outcome. An integral part of nursing assessment is first of all listening carefully and focusing on the patient. Most patients know what they need. In LTC, some may present differently because of their severe functional decline and cognitive losses. In turn, the nurse, nurse practitioner, or physician may wrongly assume that older patients do not experience pain like their younger counterparts, or that they need very small doses of medication.

Bruckenthal writes about the need to return to basics with assessment of pain in older patients. "Pain *in patients older than 65 years of age is significantly undertreated and misunderstood.*"[18] Why does this happen, and what are the barriers to treatment? One barrier to adequate pain management is how effectively we assess their pain. As discussed earlier, many nursing home patients cannot speak to us and cannot tell us what is wrong. The patient is also sick, tired, and often depressed. This is an important point to remember. An assessment must be comprehensive without being too long and tiring to the already fatigued patient. It includes several phases in an order or sequence. A nurse should have some "rules" to go by, and one of these should address the need to allow the patient to talk for the first 5 minutes about where the pain is, what specifically is hurting, and why the patient is so distressed. The first 5 minutes of focused listening and sitting down at eye level with the patient give a nurse important information about the patient. The assessment should then be directed to filling in informational gaps in the database; the nurse begins to ask direct questions with a problem-oriented or focused assessment. An assessment should be brief but thorough. The nurse should be able to leave the patient within 10 minutes and get an order or prepare the medication.

One should remember that when a person is very ill, much of the world is already closed off. It is our job to open new doors.

Bruckenthal writes about "a review of the basics."[18] The format for a focused history and physical examination should be followed,[19] and details should be presented to guide the staff nurses, the physicians, and the nurse practitioners as they review nursing notes. The chart and medication record are integral to a thorough pain assessment. In nursing homes, we do not use the rating scales as much as is done in other areas, such as hospitals, clinics, and home care. The reason is that many of our residents are cognitively impaired and cannot interpret the scales. Individual self-reports are most reliable, but it is different for many residents in nursing homes. The point is that we can still get a reliable assessment of pain. These are, however, a few of the reasons why, as Bruckenthal writes, residents in LTC, the old, the most frail, the disabled, and the functionally compromised are undermedicated and undertreated for their pain.[18]

Once an assessment is complete and the nurse calls me regarding medication, we plan together, and the chart is at the desk for informational purposes. We develop a plan based on diagnosis, current medications, age, and renal function. Age should not matter with reasonable dosing, if the patient has good renal function. It is more worrisome to have a younger patient with poor renal function. Common medications in the nursing home are Vicodin, oxycodone, Percocet, and hydromorphone (Dilaudid). Long-acting medications are oxycodone (OxyContin) and MS Contin. The fast-acting morphine derivatives such as oxycodone (OxyFast) provide the quickest relief.

In case of a urinary tract infection, the next question I ask is about allergies or sensitivities. The order is read back and the patient is medicated. I usually ask for an update regarding pain relief and how the patient is doing. Outcomes are always indicated with pain medications; they are often difficult to determine in nursing home settings.

What follows is the case of my good friend. I am, in presenting it here, honoring her and her presence in my life.

A 50-year-old with metastatic breast cancer

"Mo" was a 50-year-old woman with breast cancer and metastases to the bone, liver, and brain. She had diabetes and multiple comorbid conditions. She was divorced and lived alone. She had a supportive extended family. She had some good friends. She had a proxy and detailed advanced directive. She was alert and oriented until the last days of her illness. She called me the day of her diagnosis and said, "I have metastasis to the brain. They cannot do surgery. It is too far gone." She stopped eating and her condition deteriorated over several months; there was no option for surgery and hospice was called in at month 2. It was the holidays and her room was filled with flowers. There was neither happiness nor Christmas spirit. The hospice social worker read to her for long periods of time. Sometimes I sat there, with eyes closed, and allowed her voice to drift through my mind. Mo loved being read to.

She was sad, depressed, and angry at having to leave a life where there was so much left to do. Her lab test results were deteriorating and her renal function became more compromised. An indwelling Foley catheter was put in for comfort and to protect her skin. Her medications were Roxanol, Ativan, Levsin, and acetaminophen suppository for fever. All routine oral medications were discontinued. Her Roxanol was started at 5 mg every 4 hours as needed—it was next changed to a schedule with 5 mg every 4 hours around the clock with 2 mg every 1 to 2 hours as needed. It was again increased in a few days to Roxanol 5 mg every 1 to 2 hours as needed for pain, respiratory distress, and tachypnea. The scheduled dose was increased at that time to 10 mg every 4 hours around the clock. Scheduled doses of Roxanol should be titrated upward along with breakthrough doses. Each patient is unique with regard to symptom burden and pain control. Ativan was changed from as-needed to scheduled dosing and an acetaminophen suppository was given for fever. Mo was tough, she didn't want to let go, and it took her several weeks to leave us. Oxygen at 2 to 4 L/min was added and as time passed, it became more difficult to arouse her. Her eyes were closed most of the time. Her illness and depression precluded any engagement with life. She died in the nursing home quietly and pain-free 2 weeks later with a friend at her side. I was that friend.

Although I have cared for many dying patients over the years, it was different this time. She was my friend.

It is cases such as Mo's that evoke much discussion among nurses, family, and providers. In practice, end-of-life actions are on a continuum that stays much the same from diagnosis to active dying. Sprung and Ledoux write: "end-of-life medical actions form a continuum from aggressive resuscitation to active euthanasia, and the dividing lines between different actions are not always easy to define."[19] There are similarities across patient experiences. Letting go is not easy for the patient or family. Small rituals and a sense that certain measures are common to the dying allow the family and the nurse to "draw their line" and say, "Is this a relief of suffering from which there is no longer any respite, or, is this hastening a death?"

Sprung's work was in intensive care units, but the systematic progression of tasks with the sick is dependent on opioids and other medications, in appropriate but larger doses across settings. Pain management with opioids is a powerful intervention designed to relieve suffering at the end of life.[20,21]

A PHYSICIAN SPEAKS ON OPIOIDS, THE TREATMENT OF PAIN, AND COMPASSIONATE CARE

I graduated from the University of Madras, Madras, India. My residency was at the University of Health Sciences at Chicago Medical School, Chicago, followed by a research fellowship at Tufts New England Medical Center. It was chance and serendipity that as a junior member of an internal medical practice, more than 15 years ago, I was introduced to LTC. By applying the good "doctoring" that people call palliative care, we were able to provide quality outcomes for many frail elderly patients. I then obtained my Certified Medical Director (CMD) certification in LTC.

Geriatrics led me to hospice and palliative medicine; both concepts were part of a philosophy that I had practiced earlier. Total care is more than physical care and includes the body, mind, and soul. Modern medicine, despite its technological prowess, has failed to provide the most frail and vulnerable of older adults the care they require and deserve.

There is no greater reward in medicine than that of caring for the frail elderly or helping the dying. Through compassionate care, we give them a voice.

Pain is common in the LTC setting. As many as 80% of LTC patients have at least one condition associated with pain. The prevalence of pain varies among LTC facilities. One study using the minimum data set (MDS) showed a prevalence of pain among residents of LTC facilities that ranged from 0% to 55%; another study based on MDS data reported that persistent pain affected 49% of residents. Although disorders that can cause pain become more common with increasing age, pain itself is not a normal part of aging.

At the end of life, 60% to 90% of children report pain. Of patients with non-cancer diagnoses (eg, congestive heart failure, cirrhosis), more than 40% experience severe pain within days of death. A 2007 meta-analysis found prevalence of pain in 64% of patients with metastatic or advanced-stage cancer; more than one-third rate this pain as moderate to severe. Many dying patients experience what has been termed "total pain," a concept based on the recognition that pain is an integrated biopsychosocial and existential construct, not simply a sensory experience, and it can result in all-encompassing suffering. The 4 components are physical pain (usually from multiple sources), emotional or psychic pain, social or interpersonal pain, and spiritual or existential pain. Although physical pain was the most common source of suffering, all 4 components listed were significant sources of suffering.

TREATMENT OF PAIN

Effective treatment of pain depends on thorough assessment and specific interventions designed to relieve each type of pain. Most physical pain can be managed with relatively simple techniques, but individualized treatments and adequate medication dosages are required for effective control.

General Guidelines

Follow the World Health Organization (WHO) steps for titrating oral pharmacologic therapy.[22,23]

- Calculate accurate oral and parenteral opioid equivalents.
- Improve compliance by dispelling misconceptions about opioid therapy, and make the opioid regimen as simple to use as possible.
- Use effective starting dosages, and titrate upward as needed.
- Use appropriate adjuvant drugs to treat each type of pain.
- Prevent and treat anticipated problems, such as constipation and sedation.
- Incorporate nonpharmacologic methods, such as distraction and relaxation.

The WHO recommends a simple and effective 3-step approach:

Step 1: When there is mild pain, an acetominophen, a nonsteroidal antiinflammatory drug (NSAID), or another adjuvant analgesic may be used to control the pain.

Step 2: When pain persists, increases, or presents as mild to moderate, step 2 suggests the addition of low-potency opioids, such as codeine or a low dose of a stronger opioid, such as morphine. At step 2, fixed-dose combinations of an opioid with acetaminophen are often used because combining the drugs sometimes provides added analgesia. When higher doses are needed, separate dosage forms of the opioids and nonopioids are used to avoid toxic effects of high-dose acetaminophen and NSAIDs. Medications for persistent pain are administered on an around-the-clock basis, with additional doses as needed to control breakthrough pain.

Step 3: When pain persists, increases, or initially presents as moderate to severe, opioids such as morphine, hydromorphone, or fentanyl are needed. Patients presenting with moderate to severe pain, when first seen by a clinician, are usually started at step 2 or 3.

Climbing each step is not necessary. Severe pain mandates the immediate use of opioids for moderate-to-severe pain without progressing sequentially from steps 1 to 3. According to the basic principles of the WHO ladder, pain medications should be given by mouth, if possible:

- around the clock for continuous pain
- according to the ladder
- tailored to the individual
- with attention to detail

Misconceptions About Opioids

Many physicians are reluctant to prescribe opioids because of misconceptions about their effects. Nurses may be reluctant to administer morphine for the same reasons. Similarly patients and their family caregivers may have strong negative feelings about opioid analgesics. Health care professionals must be knowledgeable to avoid reinforcing fears and to dispel concerns that interfere with safe and effective prescribing.

- Opioids rarely cause respiratory depression
- Opioids rarely cause addiction
- Opioids rarely cause rapid tolerance
- Opioids rarely cause death
- Opioids do not have a narrow effective dosage range
- Opioids are not ineffective by mouth
- Opioids rarely cause nausea
- Opioids rarely cause euphoria

There is no ceiling or maximal recommended opioid dose. Dosages as high as several hundred milligrams every 4 hours may be needed to relieve severe pain. Additional opioid doses referred to as "breakthrough doses" are sometimes needed to boost basal analgesia. Patients' adherence to opioid treatment improves when health care providers take time to listen carefully to the patient's and family's concerns.

Effective control of pain requires continued reassessment of total pain. Nurses and physicians require expert assessment skills and an ability to listen to what the patient or family has to say.

SUMMARY

Pain has a human, thus universal, context. We echo Sontag's poignant reminder that each of us will one day, some sooner, some later, enter that "other kingdom of the sick."[2] Clinicians who care will be mitigating some of the pain. Educators must reach out to nursing homes with programs that will significantly improve the knowledge base of staff and bring best practice to LTC residents, eliminating care disparities and structural deficiencies in the LTC system.

REFERENCES

1. Graboys T. Life in the balance. A physician's memoir of life, love and loss with Parkinson's disease and dementia. New York: Union Square Press; 2008 [Division of Sterling Publishing].
2. Sontag S. Illness as metaphor. New York: Farrar Strauss and Giroux; 1978.
3. Ferrell B. Ethical perspectives on pain and suffering. Pain Manag Nurs 2005;6(3): 83–90. Available at: www.medscape.com. Accessed March 14, 2009.
4. Kane RL, Kane RA. A nursing home in your future. N Engl J Med 1991;324:627–9.
5. Kemper P, Murtaugh CM. Lifetime use of nursing home. N Engl J Med 1991;324: 595–600.
6. Reinhard S, Young H. The nursing workforce in long term care. Clinics; 44(2) in press.
7. Beers M, editor. The Merck manual of geriatrics. 3rd edition. Rahway (NJ): Merck Publishing; 2000.
8. Kenen J. The new specialty in cancer care. Cure 2008.
9. Wetle T, Teno J, Shield R, et al. End of life in nursing homes: experiences and policy recommendations. AARP Policy Report 2004; ii, iii.
10. Libretto S. Use of transdermal fentanyl in patients with continuous non-malignant pain. Clin Drug Investig 2002;22(7):473–83. Available at: www.medscape.com. Accessed March 24, 2009.
11. Glajchen M. Chronic pain: treatment barriers and strategies for clinical practice. J Am Board Fam Pract 2001;14(3):178–83. Available at: www.medscape.com. Accessed March 14, 2009.
12. McCarberg B. Realistic levels of pain relief. Therapeutic opioid regimen. Cancer Control 2000;7(2):132–41. Available at: www.medscape.com. Accessed March 14, 2009.
13. Mitchell SL, Teno JM, Intrator O, et al. Decisions to forgo hospitalization in advanced dementia: a nationwide study. J Am Geriatr Soc 2007;55:684–91.
14. Casarett D, Karlawish J, Knashawn M, et al. Improving the use of hospice services in nursing homes; a randomized controlled trial. JAMA 2005;294:211–7.
15. Hutt E, Buffum M, Fink R, et al. Optimizing pain management in long-term care residents. Geriatrics and Aging 2007;10(8):523–7. Available at: www.medscape.com. Accessed March 14, 2009.
16. Angell M. Don't blame the sick. Boston Globe. February, 2007 [Editorial].
17. McCaffrey M, Passero C. Pain: clinical manual. St. Louis (MO): Mosby; 1999.
18. Bruckenthal P, D'Arcy Y. Assessment and management of pain in older adults: a review of the basics. Topics in Advanced Practice Nursing eJournal 2007; 7(1). Available at: www.medscape.com. Accessed March 14, 2009.
19. Sprung R, Grant R, Eagle KA. Lessons learned from a community hospital chest pain center. Am J Cardiol 1999;83(7):1033–7. Available at: www.medscape.com. Accessed March 14, 2009.

20. Sprung, Charles L, Didier MD, et al. Relieving suffering or intentionally hastening death: where do you draw the line? Crit Care Med 2008;36(1):8–13.
21. American Association of Hospice and Palliative Care. Available at: http://www.aahpm.org/.
22. World Health Organization. Available at: http://www.who.int/cancer/palliative/painladder/en/.
23. American Medical Directors Association. Available at: http://www.amda.com/tools/cpg/chronicpain.cfm.

Caregiver Burden: Three Voices—Three Realities

Joan F. Wright, BA[a],*, Mary E. Doherty, MSN, ANP-BC, MBA[a],
Linda G. Dumas, PhD, RN, ANP-BC[b]

KEYWORDS

- Alzheimer's • Caregiving • Caregiver • Caregiver burden
- Caregiver stress • Dementia • Early onset • Family caregiver

ROSEMARY DONOVAN WRIGHT (BY JOAN WRIGHT)

Family caregiving is neither a career choice nor a role for which one can prepare, yet nearly 45 million Americans are presently engaged in caring for a loved one. Nearly 60% of family caregivers are women and 43% are more than 50 years old.[1] Of those family caregivers caring for seniors, 30% are themselves aged 65 years or older and 15% are between the ages of 45 to 54 years.[2] Seventeen percent of family caregivers provide 40 hours or more of care a week.[1]

Within the realm of family caregiving, some 9.8 million caregivers are caring for a loved one with Alzheimer's disease, providing 8.4 billion hours of care in 2007. Reflecting all family caregivers, approximately 60% of Alzheimer's caregivers are female relatives (wives, daughters, daughters-in-law, granddaughters). The average age of the Alzheimer's caregiver is 48 years.[3]

How and why they become caregivers is largely rooted in the relationship they share with the loved one for whom they care. For some it was a choice, for others a default position. But most agree it is indeed an act of love even though it is one that most caregivers never imagined having to fulfill.

The caregiver has no "care map" to lead the way. Articles, books, and support groups provide guidance but every caregiver's journey is a singular undertaking complete with its own set of entanglements, consequences, and perplexities. It is anything but simple; its effects are enduring and complex.

The emotional, physical, and financial impact of undertaking such a challenge creates added health concerns for an already overtaxed system. Researchers calculate the financial savings attained by unpaid family caregivers at approximately

[a] Norwell Visiting Nurse Association and Hospice, 91 Longwater Circle, Norwell, MA 02061, USA
[b] College of Nursing and Health Sciences, University of Massachusetts Boston, 100 Morrissey Boulevard, Boston, MA 02125, USA
* Corresponding author.
E-mail address: jwright@nvna.org (J.F. Wright).

Nurs Clin N Am 44 (2009) 209–221
doi:10.1016/j.cnur.2009.03.002
0029-6465/09/$ – see front matter © 2009 Elsevier Inc. All rights reserved.

$375 billion in 2007,[1] 3 times higher than spending on Medicaid home care and community-based services, and exceeding every state's spending on Medicaid long-term care countrywide. But at what cost to the caregiver? The extenuating costs and consequences of caregiving have yet to be studied and analyzed. For example, what are the financial consequences on the caregiver's health, undoubtedly affected by the emotional and physical drain of caregiving, and where do such costs fall within the health care delivery system? With 1 in 5 adults involved in family caregiving,[1] and projected demographics suggesting that these figures will increase dramatically, there is an obvious need to look beyond the front lines of caregiving expenses (ie, financial, emotional, and physical), and into the parallel levels of costs.

For example, 1 in 10 caregivers report that their own physical health has worsened due to caregiving.[4] Chronic conditions such as heart disease, cancer, diabetes, and arthritis are reported by caregivers at nearly twice the rate of noncaregivers.[5] Neglect of one's own personal health is far more prominent among family caregivers, with more than half (55%) admitting to missing doctors' appointments.[6]

The impact of caregiving on the caregiver's employment is also significant, particularly because 48% of family caregivers are employed full-time, with 11% holding part-time jobs.[1] In one study of family caregivers in which 57% were employed either full- or part-time, 66% admitted to having to leave early, arrive late, or take time off because of the caregiving; 18% needed to take a leave of absence and 13% had to reduce their hours. Eight percent had to turn down promotions and another 8% had to quit work all together due to caregiving obligations.[7]

Thirty-nine percent of Alzheimer's caregivers are engaged in active caregiving for 1 to 4 years, and the slow progression of Alzheimer's disease often extends the caregiving process even longer. The average duration for the Alzheimer's caregiver is 4.3 years[1] but 32% of family caregivers provide care for 5 years or longer.[7] Such tenure in caregiving compounds the stress for the caregiver. Approximately one third of Alzheimer's caregivers report symptoms of depression. In a study of family caregivers involved in the final year of care, 59% admitted to feeling they were on duty 24/7, and 72% expressed relief when their loved one died.[8]

Family caregiving is essential—even more so as demographics move more and more toward an aging society—whereas the economic health of our own health care system becomes weaker and more overburdened. If our present health care system cannot provide adequate care for those who need it without the help of family caregivers, how can we not expect to have to rely on this invaluable source of caregiving even more so in the future? But who will help the caregiver?

Sixty-seven percent of caregivers say they need help in finding assistance or information. The most common unmet needs identified by the Alzheimer's caregiver are finding time for oneself (35%), managing emotional and physical stress (29%), and balancing work and family responsibilities (29%).[7]

In *Alzheimer's Disease Caregivers Speak Out: A Guide to Understanding, Caring and Coping*, adult children caring for their parents who have Alzheimer's disease express the lack of understanding society has for the stress and suffering of providing such care. One such caregiver writes, "I wish society understood dealing with a family member with Alzheimer's disease is much more than dealing with a person who has memory loss. It changes everything about the person. It changes all of our lives more than other people could ever imagine."[8]

Indeed it does. My own journey in caregiving began nearly 20 years ago, and as with most family caregivers, it seeped into my life slowly without my even recognizing what it was, let alone naming it. Covering a caregiver support group for a writing assignment, I listened to the stories of others and realized with surprise that they were also speaking of my life. After years of patching holes in the walls of crises around my parents' health, my role as a family caregiver had intensified when my mother, while caring for her aunt with Alzheimer's disease, began showing signs herself. My father suffered from heart disease and, overwhelmed with the noticeable decline of my mother, gratefully invited me into sharing the primary caregiver role. And so it began that all-too-fast, no-time-to-prepare roller coaster ride of Alzheimer's caregiving. In the throes of it, I grappled to find resources, support, experts who could help light the way into this abyss that we as a family were hurtling through. But the search for information and support was often as frustrating and painful as dealing with the daily issues of my mother's Alzheimer's disease. It was the mid-1990s and adult day-health programs were limited, special assisted-living communities just coming into the picture, Aricept still in test mode, and the primary drug of the time not terribly effective. Alzheimer's care quite simply had yet to become a "specialty."

My mother vowed to fight the disease, and she most certainly did in every way possible, which of course made the journey as caregiver full of challenges. Like most family caregivers, I was unprepared, had no clinical or psychology background, and thus was a novice at interpreting my mother's symptoms and behavior. I researched journals and articles, reached out to neurologists and psychiatrists, cruised the Alzheimer's Association Web site and helpline to find answers, techniques, or just a clue. How do you respond to your mother asking to go home as she sits on her couch in her own home? What do you do when she is convinced there are squirrels all over her bed or the man lying in bed with her (her husband) is a stranger? How do you comfort her when she holds her head and cries that she hates losing her mind? When do you allow yourself to cross the line and become your parent's parent?

These are the dilemmas faced by Alzheimer's caregivers every day. Caregiving in Alzheimer's disease goes well beyond personal care and medication management. It involves walking a tightrope to preserve a loved one's dignity while keeping them safe, and carrying the burden of critically, yet compassionately, responding to the challenges and conflicts they present as they lose their ability to process life.

All too often, family caregivers operate under the radar in health care delivery and go unnoticed and unheard. It is imperative to open the doors to these men and women, hear their stories, respect the significance of their journeys, and learn from their experiences.

Learning to Speak Alzheimer's[9] is a textbook for caregivers, written by Joanne Koenig-Coste, an Alzheimer's professional who literally came up from the ranks by caring for her husband with dementia. She illustrates the painful and often brutal realities of the disease through sharing her actual experiences, punctuated with compassion and much-needed humor. Most importantly, her factual accounts give caregivers guidance, direction, and practical tools to deal with their own situations.

Other books have been published recently giving an inside look at the person with Alzheimer's disease as well as the caregiver. A common "haunt" of the family caregiver is trying to discern what the loved one is feeling and thinking. Hearing the voices of individuals with Alzheimer's disease helps caregivers work through the puzzles of this disease. *Still Alice*[10] is an extraordinary and eloquent story that enables readers to see the progression of dementia through the eyes of a 50-year-old professor who developed early onset Alzheimer's disease. Similarly, Richard Taylor[11] shares a brutally honest look at his own progression into Alzheimer's disease in *Alzheimer's from the Inside Out*.

My own quest for information, tips, and guidance led me to dedicate my career to helping caregivers find the necessary support and help, and I have been fortunate to do so as a cofacilitator of Alzheimer's caregiver support groups. Practical tools are what caregivers need in daily life. In fact, it is the primary request of everyone attending Alzheimer's caregiver support groups. "How do I . . .?" "What works?" is what they ask. Their craving for solutions can be assuaged with the anecdotes and stories shared by fellow caregivers. They become lifelines for each other in a way that science and medicine cannot. The survival, and often, the success, of caregivers is dependent on hearing from other caregivers who have been there in the same scenarios and who have come out the other side to tell their stories. Here are 2 such voices.

DANIEL EDWARD DOHERTY (BY MEG DOHERTY)

Early onset Alzheimer's disease is considered the "new face" of Alzheimer's disease affecting from 250,000 to 500,000 Americans under the age of 65 years, in the prime of their lives. It has been described as a "creeping crisis" and there are several issues that are specific to younger persons diagnosed with early onset Alzheimer's disease (EAOD) that are generally not considerations for the type of Alzheimer's disease found in older individuals. "Although the memory loss and mental confusion the disease causes is devastating at any age, it presents a different set of challenges for people with early onset Alzheimer's and their families."[12] The clinical presentation is different. Usually these individuals are still working. It is more common for job performance to decline and be noticed by supervisors or coworkers, and it is also common for the person to be unaware of changes. Initially the symptoms can be subtle, rather than frank "forgetting," and are often characterized as anxiety, depression, mood changes, or other neurologic diseases. According to the Alzheimer's Association's recent report on early onset dementia, the time lapse between seeking medical help and obtaining a diagnosis and treatment can be significant, in some cases up to a year for a variety of reasons: Dementia is not typically associated with a younger person or the physician may be in denial of or uncomfortable with such a devastating diagnosis; the patient or family members may not be reporting accurately or may be under-reporting or fearful of the full disclosure and extent of symptoms; the symptom patterns can mimic other diseases and may not be as concrete as those seen in the older person with a diagnosis of probable dementia; the situation just does not fit the picture by age or symptoms. It is also common for a magnetic resonance imaging (MRI) scan to be negative initially in younger persons. One person interviewed in the study said: "I never saw a doctor so disappointed to tell someone they *didn't* have a brain tumor."[13] The report identified several themes of concern articulated by participants who were younger persons diagnosed with dementia.

Difficulties Obtaining an Accurate Diagnosis

Age bias is a major barrier to diagnosis and testing.

The Availability of/Access to Available Medications and Treatments

There is a lack of local professional knowledge about new drugs/products and potential research activities. Affordability is an issue because many younger persons have lost their job and do not have adequate insurance coverage; out of pocket costs may make newer medications impossible to afford. Always looking for new products.

Participation in Research Projects

Participation can be hindered because research projects are more focused on persons more than 65 years. Although the age limit has been lowered to 55 years in the past few years, the participants want equal opportunity for all persons with EOAD, regardless of age.

Coping with Changes in Functional Ability

They expressed fear of losing independence and do not want the people around them to disempower them; they want to be able to function independently as long as possible and are frustrated when people attempt to talk for them, and do things for them without asking. Some persons diagnosed with EOAD do not realize, however, that there is anything wrong with how they are doing things, overestimating their abilities.

Changes in Roles Professionally and Personally

Both genders may have spent their whole life working and now suddenly that is gone; work may have been their persona. Some persons continue working with adjustments, and this seems to be what persons would prefer to do. Most do not have this option and have to leave their job. One third of people diagnosed with EOAD do not have health insurance. There is loss of income, perhaps preparation for retirement is not complete; long-term care insurance arrangements may not have been made or even considered at this age. Many people leave their job before there is a diagnosis; let go for poor performance. This situation can be financially devastating; children are typically still dependent. Several interpersonal role changes occur; the loss of role of mother, father, spouse, family, and friends. Participants were vocal about these changes, including the stigma experienced the minute the diagnosis is revealed; speaking about friends and family members treating them as though they had suddenly become "invisible," talking around and about them as though they were not there, once the diagnosis was made known. They also spoke about being left out of decision making at home, even though their disease was not at the point that this would be a problem.

Safety Issues, Including Driving

Driving was a huge issue, as it is equated with independence; several participants stated that "they would drive anyway," others discussed how they would arrange transportation, once they could no longer drive.

Care and Support Availability in the Community

Most persons felt that the availability of supportive care for a younger person with Alzheimer's disease was not available or appropriate for age, that care is much more focused on activities for older persons; there were no community services addressing the support and educational needs of this younger subset of patients. Participants felt there should be a direct connection to the local Alzheimer's Chapter from the doctor's office and information on how to access community support.

Keeping Active and Socially Accepted

Younger persons with Alzheimer's disease wanted to be included, needed, and wanted. Most recognized that, unlike the person who had been retired for a while, they were suddenly forced into retirement and were at home with little companionship of persons their age. They wanted to be cared about and, most of all, wanted to remain useful in some way.

For the past 5 years, EOAD has dominated every waking moment of the lives of my family; it has pilfered our future (in every way) as a couple and as a family, and while it kills the brain of my husband, it eats away at the heart of each one of us. It is an unforgiving disease, the long good bye that can last for years. Just a few years ago, there was little written about younger persons with Alzheimer's disease. The purpose of sharing our personal journey is to educate and raise awareness of the unique issues facing younger persons diagnosed with Alzheimer's disease and their families.

Well known author Gail Sheehy[14] recently began drafting her next book on the AARP (formerly American Association of Retired Persons) Web site about the journey of caregiving: *Turnings in the Labyrinth of Caregiving*. She describes the stages in this maze as Shock and Mobilization, the New Normal, Boomerang, Playing God, I Can't Do This Anymore!, and Circle of Care. Although we have not experienced all of Sheehy's stages, I can certainly identify with her framework to tell our story: I think we are somewhere between Boomerang and Playing God!

Shock and Mobilization

Hearing the actual diagnosis of Alzheimer's disease was devastating, even though, as a Nurse Practitioner with many years of experience, I saw some clues along the way— Danny's initial profound weight loss, myoclonus, and extreme anxiety, for example. I had suspicions that there was something wrong, but at least initially, I never considered Alzheimer's disease in my 55-year-old husband. First, I believed Danny was experiencing depressive anxiety. His job was changing and he had to take a 3-day licensing examination (which he passed). He agreed to see a psychotherapist, who, in retrospect, after several sessions, raised the first possibility that this may be a "pre-dementia" syndrome. Like me, he just couldn't put his finger on what was going on. But the seed had been planted, and I began what I call my vigilance. What else could it be? The Internet was going morning, noon, and night: tumor, exotic disease (he had been in Africa when he developed the weight loss), another neurologic disease, how about a psychiatric disorder (at least there were medications for that). We took trips to the nature food store: vitamins, CoQ10, Ginko, SAMe. My thoughts started swirling, if this is Alzheimer's disease, he will have to take early retirement, what about our finances, our 2 kids in college, how would I take care of all this and still keep my full-time job, what to do with our rental property, and dealing with my father's illness and death in our home in the midst of all this? What about the future we had planned for ourselves, and how would we fit in all those trips we had promised to take, before everything went downhill? Before the actual testing and diagnosis, I had to come to the realization that our lifestyle would change drastically and that something was just not right!

When the diagnosis was finally made, I cried all the way home from Boston, even though I had known this was a possibility. I thought to myself, is this really how it is going to end? My husband, on the other hand, spent the whole time trying to comfort me, saying things would be okay. And they were for a while, until he admitted to me a few days later, that he had been thinking of harming himself. He was prescribed an antidepressant as well as Aricept and Namenda. My husband had never taken more than an aspirin in his life and had never been sick.

Mobilization manifested itself by my googling specialists, searching the country for cures, desperate for any hope of any kind and trying to find out everything available regarding younger people with a diagnosis of Alzheimer's disease. It took over my life, and still does, but in a different way now. Still trying to maintain a normal life for my kids and my husband as we dealt with this diagnosis was particularly challenging as I uncovered more and more conflicting and confusing information, even for a professional in the field. I was so focused on keeping my husband in the loop with decision-making and socially, and how to prevent him from dwelling on the future of the disease, I really was not at all thinking about the 24-hour supervision and physical care I would be facing down the line. At one point I told him, "You're not getting away with this, we're going to Europe." Although I am sure he enjoyed himself, although he cannot remember it now, it provided me with something to remember and helped us fulfill at least one small piece of the future we had planned.

Initially we agreed to keep this a private matter because we did not want to experience the stigma and isolation that we both felt would be coming. I assured him that I would leave no stone unturned in terms of new treatments and experimental protocols. When he was accepted into a clinical trial, we were both extremely hopeful and really believed in some distorted sense that "we" could beat this. We would do everything right and we would do anything that made sense; if there was a window of hope, we would have gladly done anything. For the clinical protocol we needed to discuss the risks, which included stroke and encephalopathy. Danny's brave response was, "I have nothing to lose; I already have a death sentence."

The shock and mobilization phase for us continues, and will continue to blend into the other phases as new and different experiences crop up along the way; this was not in the plan, at least in our mid-50s! Early on Danny said that he wanted to remain useful. "All I want to do is do something useful and I want to be cared about." He was having difficulty getting words out and had developed a specific apraxia initially (he could tell a person how to do something, but motorwise he could not complete the action), and he was beginning to develop agraphia. He could still drive and to this day he has a strong sense of direction. Once people learned of the diagnosis, it became painful to watch him in a crowd and not be treated in the same manner as he had been in the past. It was like having a child that nobody wanted to play with. Even at this early stage, and I am sure out of genuine concern, I would get calls daily letting me know that my husband was seen somewhere or that he was walking to the lighthouse, which he did every day. People make the leap between diagnosis and end stage, without considering that there are people who have been diagnosed who still work, write, volunteer in the community, and so forth. Danny was still driving, doing errands, and I discovered, once he had handwriting difficulties, that he would tell the person he forgot his glasses and would ask if they could they make out the check for him. In the early onset report, a participant said, "With this disease you find out very quickly who your friends are and aren't." Family members and friends acted as though my husband was invisible, several relatives even stopped asking how he was, as though he no longer existed. It was extremely painful and hard to believe that a mere 2 years earlier, this was a man who was a chief engineer for the largest telecommunications company in the United States, and was responsible for a multimillion-dollar-a-day operation. On the other hand, my husband had some good male friends who made sure they took him golfing and out to breakfast every Saturday morning in his old neighborhood where they all grew up. This really made a difference and you could see it in him when he returned from being with them; they kept him going for several years. You face extremes; neighbors who in their efforts to help, overreact in "safeguarding" him. My husband would become frustrated and ask, "What's going on here? Is everyone in this town watching me?"

The New Normal

Sheehy's new normal phase is about the new role, its marathon features, and about living with a new uncertainty, and the realization that things will never return to the old normal. Our new roles: as Danny started to deteriorate in terms of functional abilities (dressing himself, preparing meals) and became more confused, it became apparent he would need supervision and help while I was at work. I began the search for an appropriate person and found it in my own family. My 23-year-old daughter (the light of her father's life) gave up her job, trained as a personal assistant, and cared for her father for 2 years. Neither of us wanted this, but she convinced us by saying, "No one will care for him better than I can." Our son, who was away at college, was quiet about the diagnosis and rarely spoke about it. He had no idea how upset his father was that he would not be able to help him transition into adulthood, something that every young man should be able to expect of his father. After 2 years of daily caregiving, I could see that Meaghan was emotionally drained. She could no longer watch her father declining inch by inch on a daily basis. I knew too. It was just awful. We decided that something had to change. Our son, who had graduated and lived in another state, would return to find his father more deteriorated with each visit; we lived with it every day so we were not as stunned at the decline.

Once my daughter left, it meant having to deal with a string of well meaning but, for the most part, untrained caregivers—sometimes up to 3 different people a day, adding to his confusion. Some had immature judgment skills, some spoke down to him as though he was a child, others provided activities that were totally inappropriate for his age level, and others just simply believed he would be happy watching soap operas all day. Available adult day programs in the area were filled primarily with people much older than Danny, and who suffered mixed mental health illnesses, stroke, and dementia. This did not seem the right place for him. Getting him ready for the day was taking longer and longer: up to 2 hours getting him showered, dressed, and fed breakfast, and then it took time for me to get myself ready to go to work for the day. We needed to start thinking of an alternative plan, which led us to an Alzheimer's-specific assisted-living facility. The marathon of the new normal continues: having to learn all about the differences between assisted living versus long-term care. What is and is not covered by our insurance, what services are included. This was another area of great exploration and really discovering that things are not always as they seem. "We have many young people here," said the director. Yet once again, he would be in a place where the other people were considerably older. It was as if there was no place for my husband. The only other person I knew of in the area who had EOAD, was a veteran, and he was in a VA special unit, with others his age. Danny was not a veteran. The pain and sadness around the decision-making process cannot be understated. I have taken him home twice and realized that I could not do this alone. Shortly after his admission to the assisted-living facility, he fell and broke his hip, requiring surgery. We had to hire round-the-clock private care at the hospital, which had to be paid for privately, and then to rehab in a skilled nursing facility. While at the skilled nursing facility, as lucidly as possible, Danny said to my son and me, "I never thought you'd put me in a place like this." He had not ever said that at the assisted-living facility. At the rehab, we realized quickly that there is no special care for people who are cognitively impaired, especially at such a young age, with staff expecting such a person to respond to situations in a normal way. There was no understanding whatsoever of his situation. For example, he was placed in a room with a hospice patient, who was actively dying. Imagine the confusion that this caused for him, himself being moved from his home in assisted living, to a hospital, and now to this third location in a brief period of time. We all took turns staying as much as we could and at all different times of the day for protection, while he learned to walk again. Following discharge, he came back home again for 2 weeks. It was then that I realized with profound sadness, that he did not realize he was in *his* home; his beloved greenhouse meant nothing to him, nor did the classical music he loved so much throughout our relationship. He is now back at the assisted-living facility for residents with dementia; the youngest resident there.

I believe there is some of the Boomerang and Playing God phases that Sheehy describes and that I will continue to experience these for quite some time. Danny seems happy where he is right now, but it is hard to tell exactly what he is thinking. He smiles and kisses me when I visit; we actually have a language that I am sure no one else can understand, except someone you have known so intimately and spent a lifetime with. He has an intact sense of humor, he loves a good corny joke, and is still loving those Seinfeld re-runs, laughing as though he has never seen them before.

My role as a caregiver is no longer one of physical caring, but one of advocacy and protection. In the past several years I have not had a single moment when I was not worrying or waiting for that call that something had happened, or "the other shoe has dropped." This caregiving journey is one of profound loss; it is the loss of the person you love (except that he is alive), the loss of the family you once enjoyed, the loss of hope and the future you had planned, the loss of friendships you once shared, the loss of the role of wife and partner, to one of caretaker and advocate. I have a need to let people know who my husband was, that he is still that person, and to let my children know all they can about their father, the person.

I have not reached the I Can't Do This Anymore phase, yet. I do know that despite the pain and anguish that I have experienced, I have learned so much about loss, grief, and empathy, to a level that I was not prepared for. I bring this knowledge and empathy to my practice and patients in primary care and home care with a deeper understanding and admiration for all of those who are, who have been, and will be caregivers in the future. I am equally grateful to our friends and Danny's and my colleagues who have stood by all of us on this journey.

ELEANOR BARBARA DUMAS (BY LINDA DUMAS)

I begin here with Ms Wright's comment that there is no "care map" to lead the way of caregiving. It is a road, a long one for most of us, that each caregiver takes alone, even with supports, partner, and friends. When I was young, I never dreamed that I would spend 10 years of my life as my parent's caregiver. I knew it was wishful thinking but I preferred to think, as most children do, that my parents would never grow old. That said, I am certain neither parent really expected the frailty, illness, and functional decline that occurred as they aged.

My father always said, "I never feel old inside; inside, I feel like the same person I always was. It was when I looked in the mirror or tried to do something that used to be easy, that I knew life was moving at fast forward."

Caring for them was a journey that changed me, that connected me a little more with my spirituality and that showed me I had the resilience to do what came next, to share the sadness and inevitable outcome with my friends. Caregiving also left me a better human being.

Ms Wright framed it well as she set the tone and gave substance to the concept of caregiving, and caregiver burden. We are three voices, Joan, Meg, and I. We tell our stories from 3 "realities," each with our own background, spiritual/religious connections, lifestyles, and values. Here, we are a small community, sharing common ground through our individual caregiver journeys.

My experience began with my Dad. He was my mother's caregiver even when she was younger and well. She was fragile and had been through a difficult life. One day, November 23, 1993, he slipped on the floor, broke his hip, and died 3 weeks later. My mother was left alone in the apartment she had shared with her husband of 63 years. I remember coming home from the hospital the evening my father died; I went into her room and sat side by side on the bed with my mother. I told her that "Daddy" had died in the hospital. She had been to visit him and knew he was very ill. It was at this time, however, that I fully acknowledged how much she had changed in the previous year. In past months, I had attributed her volatility and flatness to depression and poor vision. When I told her about my Dad, her affect was flat, she seemed not take in what had happened, and that the man who had shouldered so many burdens was gone. She did not understand what I was telling her. After a time I felt that her early dementia was a blessing through the funeral and the subsequent dark and lonely days. I was often impatient with her, angry that she could not be more of a support to me as I grieved for my Dad.

In the year after my Dad died, my mother became forgetful and her slow descent into the world of Alzheimer's disease began. I know she knew that something frightening was happening to her. She could not verbalize it but she fought against the inevitable, long and hard, never, ever wanting to give in to the loss of independence with routine life tasks. My heart ached for her. She stayed in Springfield in a new apartment with the assistance of 2 wonderful women who grew to love her dearly, Laurie and Char. They spent all day with her and put her to bed in the evening. At that time, she was safe with Lifeline and in an older adult residence. I continued to live in Boston for the next 3 years. I became a long-distance caregiver. From December 1993 to March 9, 1996, the 2 women gave my mother love, attention, fun, and a high quality of life. She went out every day, they cooked for her, helped her to bathe, and tucked her in at night. They dressed her beautifully, took her everywhere, and sustained for her a quality of life that was more than good. I was the only daughter in a small family. Laurie and Char became sisters to me over the next 3 years. We were all her caregivers, working together to give her quality and independence for as long as possible. A lifelong friendship began for all of us: Eleanor, Laurie, Char, and I. But the Alzheimer's disease was relentless.

By the time my mother left for her first nursing home on March 9, I was paying for care 24 hours a day. Eleanor was gradually slipping into another world, a world that began to compromise her safety and her relationships with others. Laurie and Char kept a journal every day for 3 years. It was their way of communicating with each other and me. I was home at least once a week during that time. The last entries in the journal: "We don't have many more days with sweet Eleanor..". "I will miss her. I hope she is happy in her new home." The last morning before the 3 of us drove my mother to Boston to her first nursing home, the entry read: "Smile sweet Eleanor. Goodbye." And so ended the first phase of Eleanor's long walk to heaven.

A new journey had begun for both of us.

My Mom was born on Flag Day in 1911. She would be 97 now. She always liked the fact that she was born on that day. She was an only daughter, never went to college but majored in business at a local high school. Never having been to college was a major disappointment for Eleanor. She was lovely to look at and met my father on a trolley car as they rode to work at Westinghouse in Springfield. My father always said she was the "prettiest woman I ever met" and until his death in 1993, he called her his "doll." They had 2 daughters, Cheryl and me. Cheryl's death from cancer at 37 broke my mother's heart and changed her forever.

Telling and even creating a story or series of stories about the earlier years, when a loved one was young, is an important part of being a caregiver. It is sharing the biography that she can no longer tell us. As the Alzheimer's disease progressed, Eleanor lost most knowledge of her story, she lost much of her history, and who she was in relation to others, such as her daughter. Even though she did not understand, I recreated her history through stories for me and in some way for her, with pictures and words. Her room was always filled with pictures of her, my Dad, my sister, and me.

Most of the time she did not know the face in the picture that once had been so familiar.

When Eleanor entered the nursing home, life changed for both of us. Our roles changed dramatically. Few books or research focus on the life of the caregiver of a parent with Alzheimer's disease. There is no preparation for the "new job." Garity writes of caregiver burden after the nursing home placement of a parent or family member with Alzheimer's disease. In her literature review, she found only 5 qualitative studies that examined caregiver coping postnursing home placement. One of the most interesting themes was that of caregivers living with loss. Garity explored the caregiver burdens of nursing home placement and recommended more study on the effects of relocation on caregivers.[15] This theme of loss strikes me as appropriate to the situation. As a daughter, taking my mother to a nursing home for the first time, to the first of 3 nursing homes, was stressful at best. I felt guilty, sad, and worried how I would manage my jobs as a teacher and nurse and sustain a frequent presence in her new life. What I learned over the next 3 years was different as she moved to each of 3 nursing homes. There were long waiting lists in the good ones close to Boston. Urban sociologist Marc Fried, in his work on dislocation and relocation, speaks about loss and grief.[16] He called it "grieving for a lost home." As I think about his work, which I have read many times, I think of the 3 nursing homes that my mother lived in during the last 5 years of her life. He talks about losses and relocation bringing about "a fragmentation of routines, relationships and expectations." Relocation is an "alteration in that sense of continuity that is ordinarily taken for granted." It was a series of dislocations/relocations for Eleanor, who was becoming more confused and combative. On some level, I think she was grieving for her lost home. Her real home. I was grieving too.

Home was always where my parents were. As my Dad often said to me, "home is where they have to take you in when there is nowhere else to go." When I lost my Dad to death, and then my mother to Alzheimer's disease, that home was no longer there for me. I still drive by their apartment when I go to Springfield. I look up at the second floor window in the front and can see them waving goodbye at the end of my visits.

My mother's last nursing home was a community. It was a new, state-of-the-art Alzheimer's unit. I never heard the word "no" in that unit. She had a new extended family. So did I. The nurses and aides knew us well, and it felt like a home. I derived strength and sustenance from the families, especially the daughters of other residents on the unit. Eleanor was surrounded with love and appreciation for who she was, in a safe, bright environment. There was music, and meals at round tables for 6 people.

I wrote to the staff members before my mother died, to say thank you for all that they had done for Eleanor and for me. I said to them in the letter that Eleanor did not know me anymore, *but I knew her* and that was what mattered. I knew she was safe and well cared for. I fed her "friends" who could not feed themselves. Eleanor fed herself and watched me with seemingly great satisfaction that her friends were being attended to!! I grew to love her extended family, the residents, the nurses, and the aides on her unit. They made all the difference to Eleanor and to me. I told them I would always be grateful. And I am.

Caregiving has changed me and allowed me to empathize with the caregivers of the patients I look after in the nursing homes. I have learned new meanings of "community." I have learned about its ethos and morality. As I tell my students, community is indeed a sacred place. I learned to extend my heart to the folk who were such an integral part of my mother's life.

In 2000 my mother developed pneumonia and did not respond to treatment. The nurses and social worker were very supportive. As we talked I was able to make the "hard choices" and let Eleanor go.[17] As she lay dying over a few weeks, I sat next to her, often in the night, and waited. There was no more treatment, intravenous lines, medications, or food. Staff were in and out and my mother was seldom left alone. I felt loved and supported in the midst of another, a second, "worst time of my life."

After Eleanor died, I took her back to East Springfield where I had grown up. Nostalgia still grips me when I drive through that working class community where I went to school, to church, where I hung out with my teen friends and lived the first 21 years with my parents. I took Eleanor back to St Mary's Church, the church of my girlhood, where I was confirmed. I was comforted as I knew she was, in death, by the beautiful church, the words of "Danny Boy" and a small group of our closest friends.

Each of us, you and I, move through life, entering and leaving many communities. The communities that sustain us are those where we are most comfortable, feel safe, feel loved, respected, and cared for. Life is full of relocations, grieving for former homes, and places where we derived sustenance and comfort.

Words like community, family, resilience, grief, and loss are well understood by caregivers. There is a slowly growing literature on the caregiver side of the caregiver/parent dyad. As the demographics of aging drive a new paradigm for society, the concept of "community" will be at the heart of the change.

SUMMARY (BY JOAN WRIGHT)

Just as the voices of people with Alzheimer's disease are driving changes with *Principles for a Dignified Diagnosis*,[18] the voices of caregivers can also facilitate change, which is vital now and for the future. As Dr Steve Hume, coauthor of *Principles for a Dignified Diagnosis,* and himself diagnosed with EOAD at age 61 years, says, "The face of Alzheimer's has changed in recent years, and *Principles for a Dignified Diagnosis* adds a voice to that face. It is important that we not only tell clinicians we want a dignified diagnosis, but also teach them what that means. There is a lot we can learn from each other."[18] Caregivers also add a voice to the face of Alzheimer's disease, and thus play an important role in the educational process. As our 3 stories suggest, caregivers share a sense of community, a virtual one perhaps as we are stretched out across the nation, but one nonetheless that embodies our experiences, good and bad. As caregivers, we know the brutal reality of our loved ones no longer recognizing our faces, saying our names, or even being physically able to wrap their arms around us to return a hug. But we remain loyal to the love they instilled in us. Although this disease steals pieces of us from our loved ones' minds, we never lose those pieces of our loved ones from ours. They remain fully intact in our hearts, propelling us as best we can to keep them safe, comfortable, and content. In our most helpless moments, it is all we can do. We surrender hopes for anything more and fight to ensure that it is never anything less than that.

We come from different relationships, at different stages and ages in life, to this common ground of caring for loved ones. We know better than anyone the true mission of the Alzheimer's caregiver, who not only tries to preserve who their loved one still is, but honor who their loved one once was. When we are forced to surrender care to professionals and para-professionals who have only known our loved ones through the lenses of Alzheimer's disease's, we are further pierced by the awareness that they do not know the true essence of our loved ones. As caring and compassionate as these men and women may be to our loved ones, they do not know the accomplishments and significant roles our loved ones played in life before Alzheimer's disease: my mother Rosemary, who sang "Ave Maria" solo in Boston's Cathedral at the age of 19; Meg's husband Danny, who laid telephonic cables across the world undersea as chief engineer of a ship; Linda's mother Eleanor whose beauty remained through old age, and whose fierce independence defined her despite the relentless progression of her disease.

Our journey does not end when our loved one's does. Many of us find ways to continue the charge for better care for people with Alzheimer's disease, and just as importantly, their caregivers. Our roles once again morph within the journey, shifting from advocates for our loved ones to advocates for all who are still en route, and sadly, are yet to come. We rededicate our careers and practices as teachers, support group facilitators, and clinicians, travelling separate roads leading to a common place: a community of caring. Our voices cannot be silenced until the disease itself is.

REFERENCES

1. National Alliance for Caregiving and AARP. Caregiving in the US. Bethesda (MD): NAC & AARP; 2004.
2. US Department of Health and Human Services. The characteristics of long-term care users. Rockville (MD): Agency for Healthcare Research and Quality; 2001.
3. Alzheimer's Association. Alzheimer's disease facts and figures: family caregiving. [n.d.]. Alzheimer's Dement 2008;4(2):14–5.
4. Center on Aging Society. How do family caregivers fare: a closer look at their experiences. (Data Profile, Number 3). Washington, DC: Georgetown University; 2005.
5. Family Caregiver Alliance/National Center on Caregiving. Available at: www.caregiver.org. Accessed on February 19, 2009.
6. The Commonwealth Fund. Informal caregiving. [fact sheet]. New York: Health Affairs; 1999. p.182–8.
7. Alzheimer's Association and National Alliance for Caregiving. Families care: Alzheimer's caregiving in the United States. Bethesda (MD); 2004.
8. Haisman P. Alzheimer's disease caregivers speak out: a guide to understanding, caring and coping. Fort Myers (FL): Chippendale House Publishers; 1998.
9. Koenig-Coste J. Learning to speak Alzheimer's: a groundbreaking approach for everyone dealing with the disease. Boston: Mariner Books (Division of Houghton Mifflin Harcourt); 2004.
10. Genova L. Still Alice. New York: Pocket; 2009.
11. Taylor R. Alzheimer's from the inside out. Baltimore (MD): Health Professions Press; 2006.
12. Without warning: coping with early-onset Alzheimer's Disease [newsletter]. Chicago: Rush University Medical Center; 2006.
13. Alzheimer's Association. Voices of AD: a summary report on the nationwide town hall meetings for people with early onset dementia. Chicago: Author; 2008.
14. Sheehy G. Turnings in the labyrinth of caregiving. Washington, DC: AARP; 2009.
15. Garity J. Caring for a family member with Alzheimer's disease. J Gerontol Nurs 2006;32(6):39–47.
16. Fried M. Grieving for a lost home. In: Duhl L, editor. The urban condition: people and policy in the metropolis. New York: Basic Books; 1963. p. 153–8.
17. Dunn H. Hard choices for loving people. 4th edition. Herndon (VA): A&A Publishers; 2002.
18. Principles for a dignified diagnosis: new statement to medical community demands a dignified diagnosis of dementia. Alzheimer's News. February 12, 2009:1.

End-of-Life Issues: Difficult Decisions and Dealing with Grief

Beth Loomis, MDiv

KEYWORDS

• End of life • Grief • Dying • Spiritual issues

Dealing with the end of life will be the biggest challenge any one of us has to face. Even those of us who have worked with the dying are not privileged to truly know what it is like to die. We can only surmise. Nevertheless, I would like to attempt to describe some psychosocial and spiritual issues that people face as they approach the end of their lives.

Professionals who work with the dying often say, "people die as they have lived." There is some truth in this statement, yet each person's grief is unique and reflective of the narrative of his or her life.

Those of us who are caregivers, with whatever specialty we have, work with those who are near the end of their lives. In that role, we are called to listen carefully to each person's story and to put aside assumptions that require people to close their lives in a certain way. We are called to listen carefully to each individual's hopes and fears and to their physical, emotional, and spiritual needs. We are called to listen to each person as he or she makes sense of life and loss. There is no "right" or "wrong" way to approach the end of one's life.

DIFFICULT DECISIONS
Treatment Options

There are, however, some difficult choices to make. Patients and caregivers have to make decisions concerning treatment options. Some people choose to be very aggressive in their care. They want to try any curative measure and may opt to experience a great deal of discomfort in the hope of finding a cure or delaying death. Others may choose palliative care soon after a diagnosis, not wishing to suffer, even if, by so doing, their life is extended. Some patients may wish to be heavily sedated. Others may want to stay alert, even if their pain cannot be fully controlled without sedation.

Several factors influence how people make these difficult choices. Each person has a unique tolerance for discomfort and a unique drive to live. Unresolved issues, incomplete dreams, fear of losing control, and fear of the unknown can deeply influence

Mount Auburn Hospital, 330 Mount Auburn Street, Cambridge, MA 02138, USA
E-mail address: eloomis@mah.harvard.edu

Nurs Clin N Am 44 (2009) 223–231
doi:10.1016/j.cnur.2009.02.001

treatment choices. The meaning of suffering also takes on different forms in different spiritual and religious traditions. Some people opt to experience physical or emotional distress as part of their spiritual journey. Some people opt to experience distress or pain, because it makes them feel "alive." Some wish to experience no distress.

Relationships: Whom to Engage with

Another set of difficult choices facing those at the end of life centers on relationships. Most people when they are very sick do not want to engage with many family members or friends. Family members and friends will have their own needs and expectations. Choosing whom to see and what to say to each other may be a challenge. Balancing the patient's needs and those of his or her circle may become part of the professional caregiver's role. Patients and family members may wish to share certain feelings with one another, and caregivers can facilitate this conversation, but tread lightly. Many families do not feel the necessity of verbalizing their feelings or needs.[1,2]

On the other hand, some patients may experience acute loneliness, either because they do not have meaningful relationships or because they are struggling with a need to reconcile with someone else. Such a patient may need extra attention from staff and perhaps an intervention that will enable him or her to initiate reconciliation or deal with the grief of separation.

Relationships: Surrogate Decision Makers

Many patients nearing the end of their lives are still able to make their own decisions. They should be respected and given full freedom to speak for themselves. However, although some patients are still legally competent, they have lost the capacity to make a valid treatment decision in a specific situation. To be fully capable, a patient has to recognize the necessity of a decision, understand all relevant information, options, and consequences, and be able to use this information to come up with a decision reflective of his or her values. If a patient is not fully capable of making a specific decision, or if a court deems a patient incompetent, the medical staff may have to rely on a surrogate decision maker.

This gives rise to the question as to whom patients and/or their families will choose to be the patient's surrogate decision maker. The surrogate decision maker is required to make decisions that reflect the choices the patient would have made him- or herself. This is called "substituted judgment." Many patients designate a family member or friend to be their surrogate decision maker. This decision maker may be given responsibility over financial matters or, in the case of a health care proxy, medical decisions. In the case where a patient has not designated a surrogate decision maker, one can appeal to state laws to determine "next of kin."

How does a surrogate decision maker determine what a patient might want? Ideally, the patient has left some written instructions or had a discussion about his or her preferences. If both of these venues are absent, the decision maker needs to ask what the patient would want. If no surrogate decision maker is available or an answer to this question is difficult to obtain, then medical staff may have to struggle with what they think most people would want in a given situation. In such cases, an ethics consult should be requested.[3]

Relationships: Young Children

Many elders have young children in their lives who might be part of their last days. It is common for adults to try to protect young children by removing them from end-of-life care. However, they should be included, for they are often very aware of what is going on, and they should be told what is happening right away, in clear, simple language. They should not be expected to talk at length, but they should be allowed to ask questions and have those questions answered. It is important to allow children to remain children; they should not be given extra tasks or roles. They should be allowed to participate in the family's sorrow and to know that this sorrow will not last forever, but they should not be expected to grieve as adults grieve. Their feelings should be honored and not taken away with the hope of an easy fix.[4]

Children grieve in short spurts of time and may appear to be indifferent. They are not indifferent. They will often express their grief as they play. Remember that play is the language of children. A good way to bridge children's participation with an elder during end of life is to ask them if they would like to draw pictures to give to their elder or to hold on to something that once belonged to their elder.

Relationships: Being a Burden

Perhaps one of the most difficult challenges patients face at the end of their lives is the fear of being a burden.

Many people find self-esteem by being independent and self-sufficient. Many elders find the reversal of roles they are experiencing to be difficult. Many adult children find it difficult to care for their parents when the care is demanding. Resources are limited in our society, and the help people would have received generations ago from extended family and community has in many cases disappeared.

Interventions are not always easy. Sometimes a patient is helped if he or she is given permission to use a volunteer from a local senior center or church to perform tasks he or she would have delegated to a family member. Sometimes a family member does well if encouraged not to take on the whole task of caregiving. Sometimes a patient or family member needs to be encouraged to allow role reversal, recognizing that it is a part of life.[1,5] Clearly, taking care of someone at the end of his or her life causes an imbalance in everyone's life. Patients and family members can be reminded that this imbalance will not continue forever.

Relationships: Continuing Bonds

Perhaps one of the most difficult choices anyone has to make is how to say "goodbye." Historically, people have been told that they have to "let go," "find closure," and "accept" either their own death or the death of a loved one. Perhaps this expectation came out of the work that Elisabeth Kübler-Ross did in preparation for her landmark book, *On Death and Dying* (see Further Readings).[6,7] She described 5 stages that people who are dying may experience, but grief counselors have come to acknowledge that people do not grieve in stages. People also often do not "let go" or come to "acceptance" of their own death. Those who are left grieving the death of a loved one often do not "find closure" or "let go" of the person who died.[2,5]

Bonds between the living and those who have died continue forever. Patients and their family members and friends can be encouraged by this news. Patients often need to know they will be remembered. Those left behind need to know that the pain of grief softens, but they have permission to carry the person who died in their hearts forever. Caregivers can encourage family members, friends, and other staff to let patients know the impact they have made and how they will be remembered.[6]

Unresolved Business

We all have hopes, dreams, and expectations in life. As life comes to an end, unresolved hopes and dreams can come to the surface. How a person handles the unresolved aspects of his or her life affects how that person faces the last days.

Sometimes unfinished business comes in the guise of an unfinished project. I think of a carpenter who was bedbound by the time I met him, and he had an unfinished project: a crib he was making for his first grandson, which lay unfinished in his basement. He could not rest till his son came and finished making the crib.

Sometimes unfinished business lies in a broken relationship. A patient or family member needs to make amends. More often than not, one of the parties is not physically present. The person struggling with a broken relationship may need to participate in a ritual of forgiveness (such as confession) or have the opportunity to express his or her grief at not being able to reconcile.[5,6]

Sometimes unfinished business takes the form of spiritual distress. I knew a woman who had a strong set of beliefs according to which she felt she would be judged severely by God for collecting works of art that depicted various religions. She was terrified and could not experience peace until she allowed herself to practice a form of prayer that made it clear to her that God loved her.

Dealing with unfinished business means coming to terms with one's strengths and weaknesses and with one's limits and capacities. Dealing with unfinished business means being able to say that "good enough" is "good enough." Dealing with unfinished business means being able to accept the profound limits each human faces.

Not every patient, family member, or friend has the time to identify and deal with unfinished business. Medical staff can facilitate the process, however, by acknowledging that all human beings have unmet dreams. Just giving people the opportunity to talk about hopes, dreams, and accomplishments can facilitate some reconciliation.

QUESTIONS WE CAN ASK AS CAREGIVERS

It is very important as caregivers to get to know our patients. We should not be afraid to ask questions that lead us to a better understanding of a patient's spiritual and emotional resources. Some good questions might be as follows:

- Do you have any beliefs or practices that bring you comfort and about which we should know?
- What brings you comfort and peace?
- Where do you get your support?
- What gives you strength and energy?

Questions can also be framed in a general way:

- Some people need to experience a little discomfort, and others say they do not want to feel any pain. Where are you on this continuum?
- Some people like to have a lot of friends around them, and some need more privacy. What would you like?
- I have heard many people tell me what they have done in their lives that has made them proud. What do you think has made you proud? Is there anything you would have done differently?

If the patient can communicate, try to avoid questions that have simple "yes" or "no" answers. Ask open-ended questions that allow people to tell you what is on their minds.

DEALING WITH GRIEF
Some General Thoughts

Being able to deal with grief in a compassionate, wise manner is one of the greatest gifts professional caregivers can give to patients and their families. Let us consider how the word "grief" is used compared with the words "mourning" and "bereave-ment." Grief is the whole constellation of reactions to a significant loss. A person may respond to loss emotionally, physically, socially, and spiritually. Mourning is the attempt to integrate loss into one's life in such a way that one can engage in life again. One's personality, environment, and culture affect how one mourns. Clearly, one can grieve and not mourn. Bereavement is the length of time it takes to mourn. However, once a person begins to mourn the death of someone, he or she will always mourn that loss to some degree or another. The acuity of the grief just softens. In a way, once a person enters into bereavement he or she will always be in bereavement.[8]

Grief involves a person's entire life. It affects a person's emotional well-being, often spinning him or her into a roller-coaster-like experience of emotions. Grief affects a person's physical self, often displaying itself through physical symptoms. Grief affects a person's social life. People and places that used to bring a sense of comfort may no longer bring that comfort.

Grief does not sit still. It often expresses itself in unexpected times and places. Many a person has reported talking to a neighbor in the supermarket, spilling out their whole life story before they know what has happened, and choosing not to shop in that market again. Many other people have said that they were seized with unexpected grief in unexpected places, perhaps while driving their cars or in the shower. They said that grief just overcame them, without warning.

Grief is as unique as our fingertips. Each person grieves in slightly different ways. Anything goes in grief, although if someone is at risk for hurting himself or herself or another person, appropriate intervention is necessary. People are naturally hard-wired with different temperaments. Some people need to withdraw to deal with grief; others need to talk. Some people need to frame their experience abstractly; some just want concrete answers to concrete questions.[9]

Many secondary losses accompany grief. Some of these losses are symbolic; others are concrete and real. People report losing a sense of identity, self-esteem, hopes, and dreams. These losses apply both to people who are facing the end of their own lives and to family and friends left behind.

Symptoms of Grief

As stated above, grief affects many dimensions of a person's life: emotions, physical well-being, spiritual orientation, and social life. Usually, a person experiences some form of shock or denial when he or she first gets bad news. This feeling can be a numb feeling, and the person may deny that the news is really true. If a person has been sick for a long time, shock may not be as extreme as it would be if the person's health suddenly took a turn for the worse. However, sometimes it is more difficult for a person to believe the news if that person has been dealing with sickness for a long time. It is simply a hard concept to absorb that one's own life, or the life of a loved one, is going to end.

Once shock softens, people report feeling disorganization and difficulty concen-trating. Anger, guilt, regrets, and shame can also surface. As caregivers, it is important to remember that anger likes to attack anything that moves. A patient or family member may lash out in unexpected ways or at certain staff members that they feel may be more dispensable than others.

Guilt, regret, and shame all feel the same but are 3 radically different reactions to grief. Guilt comes when a person has done something to hurt someone or something and really could have prevented the act. The only way to deal with guilt is to go through an act of recompense and forgiveness. Regrets come when a person wishes he or she had done something differently, and, indeed, would have done something differently if only he or she had had more information. Regrets take the form of a double grief: grief for that which was not done as well as the consequences of that act not being done. Regrets often lead to complicated grief. Shame comes when a person gets messages that he or she should be a different person. These messages may be internal or external. People report that they feel they should not be so sad, and they should be able to function better or even be a different person. Shame requires people to closely look at who they are as persons and the expectations they have for themselves.

People who are grieving sometimes ask, "Why is this happening?" They may not be looking for answers, but they may be trying to sort out a felt injustice or a need to control cause and effect.

People may become hypersensitive to their physical belongings. A person who is dying may want to distribute his or her belongings to people he or she considers special. If, as a caregiver, you are on that list, be careful how you accept or do not accept these gifts. It may be very important to your patient that you receive something by which to remember him or her. You will have to balance this gift with the policies of your organization. You may also see family members squabbling about belongings. Sometimes, items take on sentimental value beyond their physical worth. Sometimes, sad to say, family members may be hung up on the monetary value of their family member's belongings. Try to be sensitive to the intentions behind how a person's belongings are distributed. If a family member is struggling over whether or not to keep a loved one's belongings, it is always wise to encourage them to keep the items. It is always easier to dispose in the future than reclaim.[6,9]

People who are grieving often feel hopeless, vulnerable, or anxious. They may even experience panic attacks, which is the body's way of saying it is experiencing too much stress. Many patients who are facing their last days benefit from medication to help with anxiety. Many family members also benefit from medication, but they may also benefit from exercise, eating correctly, and aides to help sleep.[10]

The Family Dynamics

Finally, a person's family, the roles different family members play, and the dynamics between family members may change. Each person in a family holds given roles. Other family members may scramble to fill those roles. If there are unresolved patterns of behavior or family members are not allowed to be fully themselves, conflict may arise. As caregivers, we need to be aware that we may be seeing only the tip of the iceberg. Family dynamics are patterns of behavior that span generations. These patterns may become accentuated during major life transitions.

For instance, every family member has certain tasks, such as making sure that each member has enough food, clothing, and shelter; making sure that these resources have been distributed evenly among the members; and making sure that division of labor and responsibility have also been distributed evenly. If there is a history in the family of one person getting all the goodies, or another person being blamed for everything that goes wrong, that injustice will surface during tense times.

Families also have the task of teaching members how to integrate change, whether it is through death or welcoming a new baby. If there has been a pattern in a family of denying change, family members may have a hard time acknowledging the upcoming losses.

Different families also have different boundaries. Some accept the intervention of strangers; some do not. Be aware of who are the gatekeepers, the guardians, and those who make certain decisions. Be aware of the different roles family members and the patient have held in their families of origin and choice. Be aware of the family rules, how grief should be handled, and what is considered important by those keeping the rules.

Sometimes Grief is Complicated

There are different factors involved that affect how a person handles grief. One's previous losses and how they were handled are often in the background. Clearly, a person's coping style, personality, and support systems all impact how he or she deals with loss. If the death could have been prevented, then the fact that it is happening may cause undue distress. Whether or not the person who is dying had a chance to fulfill his or her dreams or live a fulfilled life affects how he or she handles the last days. Acceptance by others that the loss is real and permission to express oneself through words, actions, and rituals are very important.

Sometimes people act as if a loss is not happening. In some ways, denial does play a role, and we should never take away someone's denial without offering something in substitution. Total denial, however, can lead to unresolved grief. Unresolved grief can also be manifested if people overidealize or demonize those they are grieving. Healthy grief involves seeing our own lives and the lives of those we lose for what they are: the good, bad, and ambivalent. Sometimes grief is delayed because of pressing responsibilities or issues. Clearly, if a patient is in a lot of pain or confusion, his or her grief will be affected. A family member who has huge financial, family, or work challenges may delay grief. Finally, grief can be complicated if the loss is completely unexpected. A person's psyche can become so assaulted that he or she simply cannot absorb the news. On the other hand, patients and family members often have a chance to experience anticipatory grief, which occurs when the loss is expected, and participants have a chance to grieve before the actual death itself.[11]

How to Be a Good Listener

Grief is often a very isolating experience, and so is, certainly, dying, during which you must say goodbye to everything. None of us can accurately tell a grieving or dying person that we know how he or she feels. We simply do not know how someone else feels. We can, however, be good listeners and companions on the way.

Listening well means being empathetic, not sympathetic. It means being able to put aside one's own thoughts, needs, and desires and truly leaving room for the other. It means having the capacity to walk in another's shoes, even if one has not had the same experience as the other. When we are sympathetic, we tend to react out of our own needs. We hurt, not so much because someone else hurts, but because our own hurts are triggered. When we are empathetic, we react out of recognition of the other's hurt. We do not try to fix that other person, give advice, judge, compare stories, distract, entertain, or focus on ourselves. When we are empathetic, we are able to sit with the questions that have no answers. We are able to sit with discomfort and silence. When we are empathic, we listen quietly and well.

When family members, friends, and the patient get in each other's way, we can remind them that sometimes people act out of their own needs. Sometimes, however, people have the best intentions and act out of confusion or ignorance. We can encourage people not to totally dismiss everyone who is not helpful. Some people need to be put on the shelf and reclaimed later. Often those who are dealing with grief and loss have to take the initiative to educate friends and family on how they can be helpful. This is a difficult concept to absorb when one is hurting badly.

Acknowledging the Spiritual Journey

Above all, saying goodbye to the world and all you know or losing someone significant are spiritual journeys. *A person's very soul is changed.* Many grief experts are recognizing that we all create meaning in our lives through our values, perceptions, and, many times, personal narratives. When a significant loss occurs, a person's understanding of self and relationship to the world can shift. His or her values and perceptions may deepen or shift. His or her understanding of self in the world needs to absorb the new shift in reality. He or she needs to tell a new story about life, integrating grief and loss.

Spirituality lives within the deep undercurrents of where a person finds meaning and purpose, love and connection, an understanding of what can and cannot be controlled, and hope. Sometimes a person's spirituality is clearly represented in his or her religious affiliation. Sometimes a person's spirituality does not fit into any religious tradition. Sometimes a person's spirituality is expressed in very concrete terms, as the desire to finish a project or reconcile with a friend. Sometimes a person's spirituality is expressed abstractly, as when someone yearns to understand his or her place in the sea of humanity.

We are all spiritual persons, and we all can provide spiritual support. Patients may need to know that their life has had significance and that they will be remembered. Family members and friends may need to know that they will always carry their loved one in their hearts; but an important part of mourning is learning how to live in the world without their loved one physically present.

Sometimes people express their spirituality by talking about a world beyond the one we are accustomed to seeing. Patients may talk in metaphoric language, about going on a trip, or they may talk to invisible beings in the room. People in bereavement may talk about encountering someone who has died or receiving a sign of that person's presence.

Above all, just listen. Acknowledge the normalcy of each person's grief and acknowledge that these challenges are part of the package of grief. Remember that grief may include joy and pride, not only pain. Many people benefit from specific traditional rituals that often express a person's experience when words fail. Do not hesitate to contact a chaplain or local clergy person for help.

Continued Connection

For those who are left behind, the connections with the person who has died remain intact. One never loses connection with a loved one who has died. The bereaved often report that they do not want their loved one to be forgotten; they want to continue to engage in conversation with that person, and they want to continue to be transformed by that person's presence in their lives.[11] Traditional models of mourning have encouraged the bereaved to disengage from the person who died and to engage themselves in new relationships. More recent studies have indicated that we cannot disengage from those whom we have loved and lost. When a bereaved person makes new relationships, he or she brings the old relationships into the new.

Relationships with those who have died are living relationships. They can change, evolve, and take different forms. Grief counselors often encourage the bereaved to talk to the person who died and listen to how they think their loved one would respond, to talk about the deceased to others, and to do things that represent that person in their own lives. The bereaved person needs to be encouraged to have different feelings toward the person who died throughout his or her life and to ask how knowing the person who died changed his or her life.

Knowing How to Handle One's Own Grief as a Professional Caregiver

Those of us who are professional caregivers of whatever sort are not exempt from the impact of grief. In fact, professional caregivers can experience cumulative grief as they care for many patients who grow sick and die.

We are often pressured to work hard and move on to the next task. I would encourage all professional caregivers to recognize that grief is a natural part of attachment. If professional caregivers choose to attach themselves to their patients, they also choose to grieve. Our grief is different from that of a patient's family members, and we should remember that our relationship with the patient is different. Nonetheless, we grieve.

Setting aside time to commemorate those with whom we have worked is critical. Some organizations arrange memorial services or support groups for staff. Some caregivers choose to commemorate their patients privately.

Recognize the impact of cumulative grief. We often grieve previous losses whenever a new loss occurs. As professional caregivers, we are dealing with numerous losses, and if we do not take the time to become aware of the impact this has on our lives, 1 patient's death can tip our balance.

Embrace the joy of life. We must do as much as we can to balance our professional life with fun and healthy activities that do not deal with grief and loss. Finally, be aware of your own spiritual journey: how you make meaning in life and find value in your work. If possible, do this in the community. The community is a sacred place. Remember that the reason choices are difficult is that life is deep, rich, and profound, even in the everyday.

FURTHER READINGS

Golden T. Swallowed by a snake: the gift and the masculine side of healing. 2nd edition. Los Angeles: Golden Healing Publishing LLC; 1996.
Kübler-Ross E. On death and dying. New York: Scribner Classics; 1997.
Prend AD. Transcending loss. New York: Berkley Trade; 1997.

REFERENCES

1. Doka K, Davidson J, editors. Living with grief when illness is prolonged. New York: Taylor & Francis/Hospice Foundation of America; 1997.
2. Wogrin C. Matters of life and death: finding the words to say goodbye. New York: Broadway; 2001.
3. Dunn H. Hard choices for loving people. 4th edition. Herndon (VA): A&A Publishers; 2005.
4. Grollman E, editor. Bereaved children and teens: a support guide for parents and professionals. Boston: Beacon Press; 1996.
5. Callahan M. Final gifts: understanding the special awareness, needs, and communications of the dying. New York: Bantam; 1997.
6. Klass D, Silverman P, Dickman S, editors. Continuing bonds: new understandings of grief. New York: Taylor & Francis (Series in death, education, aging and health care); 1996.
7. Kübler-Ross E. On death and dying. New York: Scribner Classics; 1969.
8. Lewis CS. A grief observed. New York: HarperCollins: HarperOne; 2001.
9. Rando T. How to go on living when someone you love dies. New York: Bantam; 1991.
10. Hickman M. Healing after loss: daily meditations for working through grief. New York: HarperCollins: Collins Living; 1994.
11. Neimeyer R. Meaning reconstruction and the experience of loss. Washington, DC: American Psychological Association; 2001.

Hospice—Organizational Perspectives

Mary E. Doherty, MSN, ANP-BC, MBA

KEYWORDS

- Hospice • End of life • Hospice team • Palliative care
- Hospice industry

The origins of hospice can be traced to early Christianity; it was a place where a religious order provided special care to people who were weary, wounded, sick, or dying. The concept of hospice was further advanced during the late 1800s, when the Irish Sisters of Charity in Dublin established St. Joseph's Hospice, which served the dying *only* and was an important model for the British hospices of the time. The modern "hospice movement" began in 1967 with the establishment of St. Christopher's Hospice in London by Dame Cicely Saunders. Her program was the first to combine traditional compassionate care with modern pain control techniques and multidisciplinary support for the dying. St. Christopher's Hospice remains the flagship of the hospice movement in England to this day.[1]

In the United States, hospice is a relatively new concept in the spectrum of currently available health care services. Two coincidental events in the late 1960s influenced the care for people in the United States who were diagnosed with an irreversible illness. Dame Saunders was invited as a visiting faculty member at Yale University School of Nursing. Yale Dean Florence Wald and her students were so inspired by her work that they developed and eventually launched the first American hospice in 1974 as a home care program in New Haven. The publication of Kübler-Ross' best-selling book, *On Death and Dying*, partially fueled the hospice movement through the 1970s.[2] *Time* magazine said of the book at the time, "It has brought death out of the darkness."[1] People in their local communities, through personal experiences and in recognition of the unmet needs of dying persons, usually with a terminal cancer diagnosis, spontaneously developed volunteer-driven hospice-type services as an alternative to the care in the existing medical system. Kübler-Ross testified before the US Senate advocating for "a compassionate approach to our mortality, which should include the support necessary to care for dying loved ones at home and the involvement of patients in decisions affecting their care."[2,3] In 1982, Congress created legislation establishing Medicare coverage, emphasizing

Visiting Nurse Association, 91 Longwater Circle, Norwell, MA 02061, USA
E-mail address: mdoherty@nvna.org

Nurs Clin N Am 44 (2009) 233–238
doi:10.1016/j.cnur.2009.02.002
0029-6465/09/$ – see front matter © 2009 Elsevier Inc. All rights reserved.

nursing.theclinics.com

hospice care within the home, and 4 years later, the Medicare Hospice Benefit was made permanent. Insurance coverage for hospice services facilitated the movement's growth from coast to coast and allowed it to evolve from volunteer-based, grassroots organizations to both for-profit and not-for-profit health care companies with paid staff and quality practices.[4]

The inclusion of improved pain and symptom management, an understanding of the problems faced by families, and a focus on research and teaching have brought the old traditions in care and caring into the present day.[5] Hospice has grown tremendously over the past 30 years, yet a variety of barriers to hospice care persist, posing problems in access to hospice care for terminally ill patients. "Too many Americans have their access to better care and services, through hospice and other forms of palliative care, blocked by a lack of information, misunderstandings, ambivalence about treatment options, unfairly restrictive governmental policies, financial limitations and other factors."[6] This article describes the current US hospice industry and the opportunities and challenges of the future.

WHAT IS HOSPICE?

Health care advocates suggest that the biggest barrier to hospice care is a basic misunderstanding about what *hospice* really means, even among health care providers.[7] Hospice is not a place, but a philosophy of care, which provides for the physical, emotional, and spiritual needs of patients nearing the end of life and of their caregivers. Hospice care involves a team-oriented approach to expert medical care, pain management, and emotional and spiritual support expressly tailored to the patient's needs and wishes. Hospice focuses on caring, not curing. At the center of hospice care is the belief that all people have the right to die pain free and with dignity.[8] The interdisciplinary team consists of the patient's personal physician; the hospice medical director; nurses; home health aides; social workers; bereavement counselors; physical, speech, or occupational therapists; and, when needed, clergy or other spiritual counselors. The team develops a care plan that meets each person's individual needs for pain management and symptom control.[8]

HOSPICE CARE IN A PLACE CALLED HOME

In 2007, for the 930,000 patients who died under hospice care, 70% of hospice care was provided in the place the patient called "home," which included 42% private residences, 23% skilled nursing facilities, and almost 6% residential facilities. Hospice care may also be provided in dedicated, free-standing hospice facilities or residences. One in 5 hospice agencies also operates a dedicated inpatient unit or residence used for short-term inpatient care when pain or symptoms become too difficult to manage at home or the caregiver needs respite time. About 19% of hospice care was provided in a hospice inpatient facility, whereas only about 10% of patients died in hospital settings that were not operated by a hospice team. When hospice care is provided in the acute care setting, nursing homes, or assisted living facilities, the care is provided by trained hospice caregivers; the facilities, services, staff, and expenses are shared but not duplicated.

There are approximately 4,700 hospice programs in the United States, and hospice care is available in all 50 states. Most are freestanding organizations (58%), followed by 21% owned by hospitals, 20% owned by home health agencies, and about 1% owned by nursing homes. Of the Medicare-certified hospice providers, the majority are not for profit (48.6%) and 4.3% are government owned and operated (by federal, state, or local governments), whereas growth of the hospice for-profit sector is advancing rapidly (47%), caring for 35% of all Medicare hospice patients.

THE "BUSINESS" OF HOSPICE

Hospice has evolved from a volunteer-driven program of care for dying cancer patients to a multimillion-dollar business. Many people are asking just how profitable the "business of hospice" needs to be, with several of the for-profit organizations being publicly held.[9] The top 5 publicly held hospice companies control 14% of the market.[10] Growth in the hospice industry has been particularly strong among for-profit hospices, despite the industry being heavily reliant on Medicare funding. "For profit corporations with better access to funding and economies of scale will be able to compete effectively against local non-profits."[10] The profit margins for the 3 major companies ranged from 6% to nearly 15% in 2006, and so far they have been able to run profitably. These results are not without controversy. In a study conducted by Bradley at the Yale School of Medicine, "patients receiving care from for-profit hospices received a narrower range of hospice services than patients who received care from not-for-profit hospices."[11] The author suggests further investigation to "better understand the impact of profit motive on patient care, particularly for vulnerable patients like the elderly and the dying."[11] Over the next 5 years, spending on hospice care will increase by 10 %, and growth will likely be by geographic region; in Arizona, Texas, and Florida, more than 40% of the deaths in patients older than 65 years happen under hospice care, whereas in 13 states, including Massachusetts, New York, and Washington, DC, hospice deaths occur in only 20% of the population.[10] According to Wharton School management professor John Kimberly,[10] hospice is a growing health care business with room for hospice programs to continue to grow into medical conditions beyond cancer. The most striking increase is the shift in the mix of people using hospice services. By 2005, cancer-related diagnoses dropped from more than 75% to only 46% of all cases, with the most prevalent noncancer diagnoses of heart disease, dementia, and lung disease.[10] Four out of 5 hospice patients are 65 years of age or older, and more than one-third of all hospice patients are 85 years of age or older. With a rapidly aging population, the number of patients aged 65 years and older is expected to grow rapidly.

DOES HOSPICE CARE PRODUCE HEALTH CARE COST SAVINGS?

Past studies indicated that in-home hospice care was a major cost savings for the Medicare program, but according to a study published in 2004 in the *Journal of Pain and Symptom Management*, hospice care reduces the costs of care for patients with many forms of cancer, such as lung cancer, but the savings are not as apparent for other diagnoses, such as dementia, chronic obstructive lung disease, and congestive heart failure. Even the savings with cancer diagnoses are challenged by new developments and refinements in palliative techniques requiring technological interventions, such as palliative radiation and expensive pharmacologic and outpatient therapies, that raise the cost of hospice care. Health care cost savings of the Medicare hospice benefit result from several factors: increase in timely admissions, increased lengths of stay, and prevention of acute care hospitalizations. Currently, 35% of those who die in hospice care are only in the program 7 days or less.[10] The change in the mix of patients served in hospice has provided the impetus to continue the study of cost effectiveness of hospice care. One key factor is that hospice decedents without cancer tend to use more intense hospital inpatient services before they enter hospice and have more expensive hospice stays.[12]

ACCESS TO HOSPICE FOR ALL AS AN OPPORTUNITY FOR REFORMING THE MANAGEMENT OF CHRONIC ILLNESS IS A CONTROVERSIAL ISSUE

The National Hospice and Palliative Care Organization estimates that in 2007, approximately 39% of all deaths in the United States were under the care of a hospice program. This means that over a million hospice-eligible persons died in the United States without the support of compassionate, supportive care. Four out of 5 hospice patients are aged 65 years or older, and more than one-third of all hospice patients are aged 85 years or older. With a rapidly aging population, the number of patients aged 65 years and older is expected to grow rapidly, and the challenge of end-of-life care will grow more serious over the next 3 decades. Some hospice experts believe that the experience of chronic disease blends gradually into the experience of dying; it is an increasingly widespread social condition that requires a social solution to prevent the social problem of "dying badly" in the United States. They believe that "Of all the existing structures and specialties in health care today, hospice has the best chance of successfully transforming itself into this chronic care social medicine of the future."[6]

Although access to hospice care is an issue for a variety of reasons, contributors to the 2003 Hastings Center Report believe that the nature and goals of the service itself need to be redefined, with a vision of hospice as a potentially new paradigm of social health care for an aging society. Hospice would have a larger mission in the future, and combined with palliative care (covering all forms of the prevention and treatment of suffering), hospice would be viewed as a subset of palliative care especially targeted to the needs of those near death, of the "chronically dying," or the "chronically terminally ill."[5] This opportunity for the future of hospice care for all could certainly be an opportunity for the American public and will require reform and change by insurers, the US government, the health care industry at every level, and society itself. Not everyone agrees, and, in fact, some critics are extremely skeptical, citing the contributors of the report for "redefining chronic illness as terminal" and rebuffing the idea of "equitable access," implying that specific age groups and conditions are being targeted as a drain on resources and so should be placed in a specific care modality. Of particular interest is the point that, as hospice case managers, chronic health programs (palliative care) when implemented within hospice, particularly in the hospital setting, will have a new role that involves influencing care received at early onset. The need for increased regulatory scrutiny would be imperative.[13]

BARRIERS AND ENABLERS OF ACCESS TO HOSPICE

Timely referrals to hospice care are of critical importance to access of services, quality of care, and cost effectiveness, and despite adequate supply of hospice programs, and nearly full insurance coverage for hospice care, less than 40% of eligible persons use the hospice benefit. Friedman and colleagues[14] conducted a study of hospice providers to determine barriers to hospice use and successful opportunities for education and partnerships. The results included the physician, the patient and family, and aspects of the hospice care system itself.

Physician barriers included the following: (1) some physicians have difficulty in accepting death and discomfort and discussing end-of-life issues; (2) physicians are educated and professionalized to cure, and they often continue to aggressively use cure-oriented treatment into the last stages of the disease; (3) physicians who view their inability to cure a patient as their own failure may view hospice as a sign that they have given up; (4) many physicians are uncomfortable with the pain management medications that are part of end-of-life care; (5) physicians who have not had training and experience do not have the skills to work comfortably with dying patients and their families; (6) physicians may have little knowledge about the benefits for terminally ill patients and how hospice reimbursement works; and (7) some physicians may be too busy to manage dying patients well, yet will not refer them, because it is not in their financial best interest.

Barriers related to patients and families were as follows: (1) discomfort with end-of-life issues is common; (2) many people associate the word *hospice* with "giving up" (this negative connotation acts as a barrier to referrals among health care professionals, patients, and families); (3) patients lack complete information or they are misinformed about hospice; (4) patients often have difficulty making the transition to hospice care; and (5) patient preference for life-sustaining treatments is common.

Finally, barriers that relate to the hospice system itself are as follows: (1) definitions of "end of life" are often too narrow; (2) the 6-months-or-less-to-live rule causes problems; (3) Medicare fraud and abuse damage the system, and investigations probing for such abuse impose burdens on organizations (even when no abuse is found); (4) finances are limited and there are coverage disparities among insurers; and (5) attitudes and assumptions (interpersonal relations) of hospice personnel can be barriers.

The authors discuss the fact that "dying patients and their families are not getting the care they need or want." However, all of these barriers offer the opportunity for hospices to provide marketing and education to physician groups, the communities they serve, and the public at large. Multiple successful education and outreach opportunities were reported by the hospice respondents participating in the study.

POLICY BARRIERS TO HOSPICE CARE ACCESS

Several other policy issues are recognized impediments to accessing hospice care. Medicare reimbursement is problematic. Milliman and Robertson reported in June 2000, "… Medicare reimbursement is not adequate to cover the costs of care for hospice patients." The recommendation, based on the shift to a more chronic terminal illness model, is to revisit the policy. The 6-month certification policy discourages physicians from referring to hospice early. Many physicians feel that they cannot accurately predict death, and they are concerned about potential fraud and abuse allegations. Another policy issue is that the patient who chooses to receive hospice care in a nursing home must make a choice between skilled nursing care or hospice care. Choosing hospice requires that the patient now pay for room and board out of their own pocket. Nursing home patients frequently forego hospice care.[15]

Data are critical to understanding the cost, use trends, and quality of hospice services; data turned into information are critical to others in understanding hospice care and its quality and financial outcomes, which in turn offers opportunity for improving access. The recent emphasis within the hospice industry on measuring hospice care quality will allow for delivering the message in objective, tangible terms: that the hospice program improves quality of life, that it manages pain and other symptoms, and that patient and family satisfaction is extremely high.

Hospice is About Living

Hospice is changing and expanding services to settings other than home. Negotiations between the patient, the family, or significant others and the hospice team are ongoing as life changes for the patient over time. Criteria for entry to hospice have been liberalized, and we honor each patient and his/her quality of life choices. Therefore, it is about living and no longer about waiting to die.

Demographics alone indicate that the hospice industry will continue to experience a healthy expansion over the next decade. The promise of very exciting partnerships and opportunities in both palliative care and hospice care in the community, in acute care, long-term care, and assisted living facilities offers new paradigms in care delivery that have promise for reforming the delivery of health care in the United States, in terms of symptom management of chronic conditions and helping patients and families learn about and actively participate in the dying process. This is an exciting period for those involved with hospice and palliative care. The recognition of the vital nature of these services will be uncovered through further evidence-based study and investigation of the costs, quality, and timing of services moving forward.

Understanding the concepts of hospice, palliative care, and end-of-life choices is important work for everyone, for we will each be at some time "a citizen in the kingdom of the sick."[16]

REFERENCES

1. Health Council of S. Florida, Inc., Hospice Foundation of America. HMEP [Hospice Medicaid Education Project] Final Report, Part I: The historical and future implications for hospice. 2002.
2. Kübler-Ross E. On death and dying. New York: Scribner; 1997.
3. Caring community hospice of Courtland. History. Available at: http://www.odyssey.net/subscribers/hospice/History.html. Accessed January 1, 2009.
4. Brief history of hospice movement. Hospice of Michigan. Available at: http://www.hom.org/movement.asp. Accessed January 1, 2009.
5. Saunders DC. Origins: international perspectives, then and now. Hosp J 1999;14(3-4):1–7.
6. Jennings B, Ryndes T, D'Onofrio C, et al. Access to hospice care: expanding boundaries, overcoming barriers. Hastings Cent Rep 2003;33(Suppl 2), Special.
7. Gazelle G. Understanding hospice—an underutilized option for life's final chapter. N Engl J Med 2007;357:321–4.
8. National Hospice and Palliative Care Organization. NHPCO facts and figures. Hospice Care in America—2007 Findings. Available at: http://www.nhpco.org/i4a/pages/cfm?pageid=3252&3252. Accessed January 24, 2009.
9. Bishop S. A hospice dilemma. The University of Southern Mississippi, School of Nursing. J Health Ethics 2008;1(2). Available at: http://www.ethicsjournal.umc.edu/ojs2/index.php/ojhe. Accessed January 24, 2009.
10. The Business of Hospice Care. University of Pennsylvania Wharton School. May 31, 2006. Available at: Knowledge@Warton:On line business journal of the Wharton School at University of Penn. http://knowledge.wharton.upenn.edu/article.cfm?articleid=1493. Accessed January 1, 2009.
11. Bradley E. Hospice care operated by for profit companies provides narrower range of services. Medical Care May 2004;42(5):432–8. Available at: http://www.opa.yale.edu/news/article_print.aspx?id=2928. Accessed January 1, 2009.
12. Tupper J. Barriers to medicare hospice utilization: a qualitative study of Maine's medicare hospice providers. Portland (ME): University of Southern Maine, Muskie School of Public Service, Institute for Health Policy; 2007.
13. Ward K. OpEd–Hospice moves to redefine chronic illness as terminal. North Country Gazette. September 26, 2006.
14. Friedman BT, Harwood MK, Shields M, et al. Barriers and enablers to hospice referrals: an expert overview. J Palliat Med 2002;5(1):73–84.
15. Christopher M, editor. Hospice care part I: A policymaker's primer on hospice care. State Initiatives In End-of-Life Care 2001;11:1–8.
16. Sontag S. Illness as metaphor. New York: Farrar, Straus & Giroux; 1977. p. 1.

Technology and Home Care: Implementing Systems to Enhance Aging in Place

Jackie Crossen-Sills, PT, PhD*, Irene Toomey, RN, MBA,
Mary E. Doherty, MSN, ANP-BC, MBA

KEYWORDS

• Technology • Home care • EMR • E-learning • Telehealth

For more than a century, local nonprofit Visiting Nurse Associations (VNAs) have transformed their organizations and have confronted whatever health care challenges their constituents have posed, in an efficient, effective, and caring manner. America's health care is in crisis. Affordability, accessibility, and quality of care are the central issues. Escalating health care costs and spending, the increasing prevalence of chronic disease and disability, and an aging population have converged as qualified resources are shrinking.[1] "While institutional care will remain a necessary part of the health care system, only home and community based care has the potential to meet this growing need in a cost-effective manner." The longstanding mission of VNAs has been to preserve the quality of life and independence for individuals by offering skilled professional care at home and a wide variety of community support services. VNAs are the experts in chronic care management, which successfully reduces expenditures for the highest-cost chronic conditions: diabetes, congestive heart failure (CHF), chronic obstructive pulmonary disease (COPD), and cancer. As millions of baby boomers retire and age, the marketplace is already beginning to develop to offer a multitude of products and services to help seniors age in place.[2]

Today's challenges for board and executive leaders of community-based, nonprofit VNAs are multiple, complex, and are reflective of the broader issues facing the US health care system. The most glaring challenges are as follows: (1) The shortage of qualified nursing and other licensed clinicians to meet the current and future demand for home health care; (2) labor, education, and health insurance costs that exceed reimbursements; shrinking reimbursements from payers and an increase in the uninsured population; (3) investment losses created by a national economic insecurity; (4) and the substantial financial investments in new technologies that will enable a more

Norwell VNA and Hospice, 91 Longwater Circle, Norwell, MA 02061, USA
* Corresponding author.
E-mail address: jcrossensills@nvna.org (J. Crossen-Sills).

efficient, effective delivery of health services, without any reimbursement mechanism. However, most of us recognize tremendous opportunity for VNAs to play a pivotal role in the solution for the long-term care of people at home, where they prefer to be cared for.[3] The national health care agenda to improve efficiencies, reduce costs, provide high-quality evidence, and performance-based care, while simultaneously meeting stricter legal and regulatory requirements, has forced home care and hospice staff to change the way they work. These pressures now require a reliance on new technologies to meet these goals. The most important question that every organization needs to consider first and foremost is "how will the patient/family benefit" from this new technology and how will the use of the new technology help ensure access to compassionate and consistent care across the continuum? The technologies identified with the most direct benefit for home health care patients are the following: point of care, telehealth, telephony, personal emergency response systems, and office automation. Secondary patient care benefits may be viewed as organization-wide clinician development tools, such as e-learning and performance management systems.

Home care by its very definition helps people to age in place. To accomplish cost-effective, outcome-driven, widespread, yet individualized, patient-focused care we require tools that will allow for the application of critical thinking and intervention skills by licensed professionals whose goals are the early identification of symptoms, prevention of hospitalizations and patient/family self-management of chronic conditions, and mastery of safety issues. Decreased costs using this technology are derived from reduced hospitalizations and emergency room visits of patients with complex, chronic health care needs, the more effective use of clinical staff, (although telehealth is not a substitute for necessary home visits), and the avoidance of nursing home placement. Industry leaders agree that telemonitoring may represent a financial solution for home health agencies despite the fact that insurers do not pay for telemonitoring. Agencies have been able to monitor patients daily and schedule visits based on patient need rather than a set schedule, while a number of studies have shown that telemonitoring has also had a positive impact on both quality and access.[4] Telemedicine is the most frequently discussed and described in conjunction with home health care technology, yet combined with the other technologies currently being used in the preparation, communication, and provision of home health care by today's VNAs, all contribute to safer, more effective, more coordinated, and cost-efficient care.

Senator Kennedy's call to action (January 29, 2009) in testimony before the US Senate: Health, Education, Labor and Pensions Committee Hearing speaks of the context and urgency of ensuring access to care that is of high quality, safe, and effective.

The overly complex and fragmented structure of our health care delivery system contributes to the lack of quality. Since our current fee-for-service system does not reimburse for coordination among health care providers, omitted or duplicative procedures, delays in care, and medical errors are common. We are losing countless opportunities for an efficient and reliable means of recording patient data and coordinating care.

The next sections describe how one nonprofit, community-based VNA implemented technologies that significantly and positively changed the delivery of home health care to the patients in their community and assisted them to achieve their organization's strategic initiatives.

The Norwell Visiting Nurse and Hospice is a free-standing, volunteer-governed, home health agency that has been providing home health care, public health, preventative care, health education, and support services to patients and families on the South Shore of Massachusetts for more than 88 years. The organization has an operating budget of $11 million and is one of the 61% of home health agencies that rely on a point-of-care technology system.[5] Rapid growth due to increased demand for home care services, regulatory documentation requirements that linked patient assessments with financial outcomes, the need for differentiation to compete for highly qualified clinicians, and a desire to be able to proactively case manage and measure clinical outcomes led the organization to automate clinical care and operations in 2003. We knew that technology had the potential to significantly change the delivery of home health care. Since then, systems have become more sophisticated in terms of functionality and can create an environment for improved outcomes, with integrated disease management programs, care planning, and reporting. Today's systems promote greater accountability and interdisciplinary communications, which ensure that the team is working together to improve patient care.[6]

ELECTRONIC DOCUMENTATION SYSTEM

Home care has traditionally taken an interdisciplinary approach to care that relies heavily on coordination and communication. This can be very difficult outside of the 4 walls of an inpatient facility. Home care clinicians in the 1990s relied on paper documentation, telephone communication, and intermittent case conferencing to coordinate patient care. It was a less than perfect system, which became more difficult as the documentation requirements grew.

In early 2003, the burden of documentation combined with problems related to efficient communication and case management was the catalyst to move from a paper-based system to electronic documentation system. This technology would enable more timely documentation and provide clinicians access to the information they needed to deliver patient care and make clinical decisions.[7] It would also provide a consistent documentation structure and legible notes, and improve accuracy. These were the obvious advantages, but we did not fully realize the power of integrated clinical and financial software systems. The benefit of an electronic documentation system would permeate our entire organization and improve operations, planning, and most importantly, patient care.

There were many considerations in the selection of a clinical software system. The major concern was how it would affect the end users, both the clinician and ultimately the patient. Involving clinicians in the process of selection and implementation was essential to a successful transition. What clinicians wanted was a system that was portable, easy to use, and one that would not impede patient (face-to-face) communication. A personal digital assistant (PDA) was selected as our point-of-care device. This small handheld device lacked some of the functionalities of a laptop computer, but it was lightweight, with a simple design, and did not place a large technological barrier between the patient and clinician. The PDA provides the clinician with access to all recent entries into the medical record. The record is integrated, and the clinicians can view the assessments of all disciplines involved in the case. Important patient information can be forwarded to other clinicians using an internal e-mail system, and alerts and reminders can be attached to specific visits. This enhanced communication facilitates effective coordination of care, provides the clinician with the confidence of "real-time" information, and potentiates optimal patient outcomes.

The role of leadership was vital to the success of the project. The clinical and support staff was assured that they would receive all the support and education needed to master the new technology. A vision of a "paper-free" organization was created and communicated to the entire agency. We were consistent and clear that everyone would learn and use the new technology; there were no exceptions.

Implementation of the electronic documentation system was simultaneously painful and exhilarating. Using a "train-the-trainer" model, the agency implementation team was taught each module and then the staff were instructed the following week. This made for a very hectic schedule. Staff members were assigned to specific groups for training. The group size was 10 to 12 clinicians with 1 instructor. By the end of the first week, we had learned some important lessons. First, our groups were too large, and second, we needed 2 instructors for each group; one to teach and another one to circulate and make sure everyone was navigating the software correctly. We also needed to offer more training sessions and be constantly available for questions throughout the day. We had multiple sessions; mornings, afternoons, and weekends. The staff selected the time and group they preferred, and eventually groups with similar learning styles emerged. We were able to successfully train staff aged 25 to 65 years with very different technical abilities and educational and clinical backgrounds during a 3-month period.

The amount of information that became immediately available to us was staggering. Suddenly we could look at patient information in real time and monitor key operational metrics and clinical and financial indices. Our overall efficiency soared, and we could finally perform trend assessment and use practices of clinicians for quality-enhancement activities, which directly improved our primary goal of improving patient care delivery and patient outcomes. For the first time, we could actually measure outcomes of care, clinically and financially.

TELEMEDICINE

The pressure to discharge patients from acute care has led to medically complex patients being cared for at home. About 75% of the nation's $2 trillion medical care costs are for individuals with chronic diseases. More than 130 million Americans have been diagnosed with at least 1 chronic condition.[1] Many have multiple and complex chronic diseases that require clinical management to prevent rehospitalization. Access to information provided us with the ability to analyze our unique patient demographics and helped us to identify factors that contributed to emergent (unplanned) emergency room visits, hospitalizations, and rehospitalizations. We learned that one-third of the patients who were rehospitalized during an episode of care went to the emergency room complaining of difficulty with breathing. The most critical period for rehospitalization was during the first 2 weeks of admission to home care. This information allowed us to examine diagnoses relating to difficulty with breathing, our current practices, and evaluate care options based on available evidence-based practices in home health care. To decrease hospitalizations, all patients with diagnoses of CHF and COPD were provided with "frontloading of services." Clinical staff members were educated about standardized assessment parameters and symptom management techniques, and care pathways were developed. Nurse specialists and advanced practice nurses worked as clinical consultants to the staff both with case review and in the home. Although this was a great start, to appreciably impact improved systems to help patients remain safely and symptom free at home, once again, we turned to technology. The question was "how we could provide clinical care and reassurance to patients with similar clinical diagnoses, teach them to manage their symptoms through education and feedback, and help them remain symptom free at home, without adding more visits and costs per episode of care?" What early clinical indicators could be detected with remote monitoring and clinical intervention?

In 2004, the agency decided to enter into the telehealth area to provide our patients with the most efficient and effective care and to promote excellence in outcomes of care. The decision to purchase or lease was difficult, because telehealth was and remains nonreimbursed by any health insurer, yet the ability to monitor patients and educate them in disease self-management was essential to preventing exacerbations and emergent care.

Of the limited remote monitoring options available at the time, we selected a telehealth solution that when placed in the home permitted transmission of patient vital signs and the ability to ask customized questions for early identification of even subtle signs and symptoms of exacerbation of the chronic illness. This technology not only allowed better symptom management but also engaged the patients in their own plan of care. [8] We quickly discovered that telemedicine was not just a remote assessment tool, but it was also a powerful patient teaching tool. This combination of technical resources, enhanced clinical expertise, and an empowered patient resulted in successful disease management and improvement in patient outcomes. Currently, we are using remote monitoring for patients with COPD, CHF, and diabetes. As we expanded and refined our program, the agency's patient hospitalization rates declined significantly. Based on Medicare (Centers for Medicare and Medicaid Services) use data, unplanned hospitalization rates have decreased by a rate of more than 10% since our implementation of telehealth. When considering the upcoming Medicare pay-for-performance implementation, clinical outcomes, including keeping patients safely at home as evidenced by hospitalization and rehospitalization rates, the use of remote monitoring of patients is an essential component of home health care delivery. The most obvious financial benefits of telehealth are the cost savings of reduced patient admissions to acute care, the cost savings to the organization in visits that are directed by need versus routinely scheduled, and the ability to provide more care (daily) to more patients at the same time.

TELEPHONY

Within the next 2 years, we realized that a very vital component of communication and integration of patient care was missing. The missing link was the timely communication with the most intimate and one of the most important members of the health care team, the home health aide (HHA). When the agency implemented the electronic documentation system, the HHA documentation remained on paper. The scheduling package for the HHAs was used, but the actual day-to-day documentation of patient visit data was filed into the remaining agency paper chart. The professional staff rarely accessed the paper chart due to the use of the PDA. We recognized the importance of standardization, improving the coordination of care and enhancing efficiencies, so once again we harnessed the potential of technology.

The options available for HHA documentation that connected with our EMD involved the telephonic recording of vital visit activities and patient data by the HHA. This telephonic platform linked into our clinical record and would allow us to meet the challenge of improving communications to all disciplines involved in the care and services of the patient. Through the patient's home telephone or the agency issued cell phone, the HHA was able to complete all aspects of the patient care note. The telephonic system allows our agency to provide more accurate and updated scheduling through real-time data. The new system notifies the HHA to changes in their schedule as the day progresses (due to patient discharges, physician appointments, cancellations, or hospitalization). It also provides GPS directions to the patient's house, a patient profile with summary information, and the name of the primary nurse. The HHA is never alone.

The telephonic system also allows the HHA to accurately check in and out of the patient's home visit. It assures accurate start and end time for the patient visit, provides accurate mileage, alerts the HHA to e-mail communications, and informs the HHA of updates/changes in the plan of care. At the time of departure from the patient's home, the HHA answers yes/no questions based on the current plan of care. This is directly entered into the electronic documentation system, and an alert can be generated to the primary nurse if any adverse changes in the patient's condition are noted during the home visit (such as a recent fall, increasing symptoms, or a change in skin status). Administratively, this HHA telephonic system allows more accurate scheduling and use of staff and payroll accuracy. It has cut administrative time in half by eliminating the review of paper day sheets and payroll entry. Even more importantly, it has now bridged the gap between the HHA and the primary nurse by improving the smooth flow of information between caregivers, ensuring the most up-to-date plan of care.

E-LEARNING

As the agency became more automated, clinicians realized that they did not need to come into the office daily to retrieve charts or materials. They began to start their workday from their home, often going directly to their first patient visit. Scheduling and providing educational programs (both mandatory compliance programs and annual competencies and on-going professional development in-services) were becoming more difficult. We were often providing programming 4 to 6 times in a given week, to ensure that all staff could participate. Attendance surveillance was very time consuming and cumbersome.

Growth demanded geographic teams. Assignment to a geographic area is often based on where the clinician resides, which improves efficiency due to limiting travel; however, it also means that with technology, clinicians no longer have to be routinely physically present at the agency. With a staff of more than 150, the challenge to identify a more efficient way to meet the orientation, annual competency, and ongoing educational needs began. A full staff survey was conducted to determine optimal days and times for in-services and training, with results indicating that there was no universal time. An e-learning solution might be an opportunity for us to provide consistent education and training online and allow clinicians the opportunity to complete the training when it was convenient for them, even from home. It was time to turn to technology again.[9,10]

We began an investigation to learn more about the various "Learning Management Systems." A hosted provider seemed like the best solution for our agency, as we were unsure of our ability to manage a server and software. This immediately honed down the choice of vendors. We wanted a system that would be user friendly for our clinicians as well as for the e-learning manager at the agency level. The project manager for this effort was a senior manager and former college professor who had experience with online course development and uploading course content. She assisted in determining a product/vendor who was affordable and who could meet our needs now and in the future. The chosen vendor allowed us to deliver course content easily; track and report learner progress; assess learning outcomes; report achievement and completion of learning tasks; and maintain employee records of completion.

Mandatory in-services for all the staff were uploaded, and it was decided to continue to offer both live and online programming to accommodate different learning styles. There was a palpable excitement throughout the agency as we approached our first online training. Brochures were created to walk each staff person through the log-on procedure, and before we knew it, the majority of the professional staff was using online learning. When there is a didactic component, the staff members are required to come in for the development of a hands-on skill, but the theoretical aspects may be completed online.

Initially, mandatory courses were implemented (Infection Control, Confidentiality, Hand washing, Emergency Preparedness, and National Patient Safety Goals). We quickly realized that our all-employee common orientation content would be a perfect fit for online training. Our courses have expanded, and there are 3 managers/senior staff who now upload programming and monitor the online programs. This was a logical and necessary step for our agency to embark on for staff convenience. The staff recognizes that the online learning is a wonderful opportunity for them, as it allows completion of online courses whenever the time is right for them. Even the board of directors participated in online learning modules to prepare for strategic planning.

In addition, in-house computer stations are set up for staff who do not have computer access at home and in need of program completion. We find that staff often use the agency computers for courses, when they are in the office waiting for a team meeting or other events. The clinicians also have access to training videos online so that if they need a refresher on a specific procedure or technique, they can review it on line before going out to see the patient.

The data we are able to capture from online training ensure staff compliance and allow managers to monitor staff progress and commitment to continuing education and training as a component of performance management. Completion of agency-mandated courses, such as annual physical assessment competencies and symptom management updates, reflects the organizational philosophy of improving patient care through lifelong learning by its clinicians. We believe that our job (management) is to enhance the workplace and improve efficiencies for our employees so that their focus is entirely on patients and patient care.

So where are we headed now? This year the Norwell VNA and Hospice will implement an online performance management system, which ties the goals of the organization with the individual performance of our employees. The technology allows for online performance appraisals by managers and staff, tracks the attainment of personal and professional goals, and helps managers and staff to actively and routinely track performance.

We are continually evaluating our current technologies/vendors against the latest available technologies that offer opportunities for keeping patients symptom free and safely at home (**Box 1**).

Box 1
Key points in home care

- Home care by its very definition helps people to age in place.
- The missing link often can be the timely communication with the home health aide.
- In 2004, the VNA decided to enter the telehealth area.
- Using a "train-the-trainer" model, the agency implementation team was taught each module and then instructed the staff.

REFERENCES

1. Visiting Nurse Associations of America. Home and community-based care: building a more effective healthcare system. Washington, DC: Visiting Nurse Associations of America; 2008.
2. Waters B. Aging in place. Home Care Technology Association of America (HCTAA Update) Available at: http://www.hctaa.org/aging.html. Accessed February 15, 2009.
3. Rintels J. An action plan for America: using technology and innovation to address our nation's critical challenges. Benton Foundation; 2008. Available at: http://www.benton.org/sites/benton.org/files/Benton_Foundation_Action_Plan.pdf.
4. Averwater BD. Technology. No place like home: telemonitoring can improve home care. Healthc Financ Manage 2005;4:46–52.
5. Fazzi R. National study on the future of technology and telehealth in home care. Northhampton (MA); 2008.
6. Coughlin J. Old Age, new technology, and future innovations in disease management and home health care. Home Health Care Manag Pract 2006;18(3): 196–207.
7. Hillestad R. Can electronic medical record systems transform health care? Potential health benefits, savings, and costs. Health Aff (Millwood) 2005;24(5):1103–17.
8. Goldfarb B. Tomorrow's technology is saving money today 2008 (April). Available at: http://www.managedcaremag.com/archives/9804/9804.telemed.shtml. Accessed February 15, 2009.
9. Clarke A. A strategic approach to developing e-learning capability for healthcare. Health Info Libr J 2005;22:33–41.
10. Cobb S. Internet continuing education for health care professionals: an integrative review. J Contin Educ Health Prof 2004;24(3):171–80.

The Challenges to Long-Term Care: A Personal Account

Frances L. Portnoy, RN, MA, MS, PhD

KEYWORDS

• Life care community • Home care • Family • Generations
• Personal account

Providing home and institutional services for the aged who can no longer care for themselves and live independently is a serious challenge to a country with wide economic, cultural, and generational differences. Planning for the future involves an intricate network of factors: not only population aging in general but also changes in family structure, availability for caregiving, early hospital discharge, and decreased length of stay, resulting in increased acuity in the population. Home care is increasingly technological, and the training and availability of a long-term care workforce is in question. These factors, in the context of rising health care and long-term care costs in a contracting economy, present problems for family, self, the private sector, and government.

To a large extent, every person as he or she ages presents a unique challenge. For new immigrants and populations who have suffered from prejudice and scarce resources, the options are limited. This is a story of how the experience of aging and the needs for long-term care assistance affect one middle-class family. Over 3 generations, there have been wide differences in expectations and experiences of aging, presenting new and differing challenges to the systems of care.

THE STORY

Sitting in my study, I can see the pictures of my family on the wall. There is my great grandmother, seated in a large chair, her head and body covered in dark cloth, her face unlined. She lived with her oldest daughter and family in Europe, until she died, untimely, in a kitchen fire. Next to her, my maternal grandmother, a European "grand dame," white-haired, wearing an elegant, black, embroidered dress and cap, dignified and aristocratic. In a round frame, my paternal grandmother dressed in more "modern" garb, who had emigrated, with my father, to the United States after World War I (WW I), stands close to her son under an imposing wall clock. All of these women

University of Massachusetts Boston, College of Nursing and Health Sciences, 100 Morrissey Boulevard, Boston, MA 02125, USA
E-mail address: frances.portnoy@umb.edu

Nurs Clin N Am 44 (2009) 247–252
doi:10.1016/j.cnur.2009.02.003
0029-6465/09/$ – see front matter © 2009 Elsevier Inc. All rights reserved.

were widowed early, raising large families by themselves. They worked hard and, by their early 60s, were "old." They fully expected to live with one of their children and help with the cooking and child care, as part of the new extended family. The children also expected that they would care for their mother (or father), for the remainder of their lives.

THE SECOND GENERATION

Thirty years ago, when my father was 87 years old, his (second) wife of 40 years died. He had emigrated to the United States as a young man, joining a brother and 2 sisters who had left Europe before WW I. He was a strong working man who spent most of his life owning and operating small grocery stores, often working 7 days a week. When he was 70 years old and urban renewal took over his store, he found a job as a cleaning man in a factory in his town. Others in the family were quite distraught, believing that such a job was beneath his dignity. But to my father, work was essential to his life and being. In his 80s, he felt strong and healthy yet was subject to some of the health problems of the aged. He had surgery for prostate cancer, for colon cancer, and suffered from several bouts of unaccountable dizziness. He remained optimistic and continued to work as a sexton in the small synagogue in his town. He also continued to live alone in his apartment in elder housing. One morning, returning from his work at the synagogue, he entered his apartment to find his glass coffee pot on the stove, burning hot, with the gas still on. This was a jolt and a shock and a moment in which he felt it was no longer safe for him to live alone. Many of his generation moved in with their children, more or less a cultural expectation. "Honor thy mother and thy father." However, for some elders this was problematic. Barbara Myerhoff,[1] in her study of Jewish elders in a California community, describes the experience of Basha, an elderly woman whose daughter was worried about her living alone and wanted her to come and live with her. Basha refuses and says "What would I do with myself there in her big house, alone all day, when the children are at work? No one to talk to, no place to walk. My daughter's husband doesn't like my cooking, so I can't even help with the meals. When I go to the bathroom at night, I'm afraid to flush, I shouldn't wake anybody up."

My father felt some of the same barriers. His children both lived a distance away, his son in another state, and he believed strongly that children had their own families and their own lives. His own life, as a religious man, would be compromised by living in a household that did not abide by the religious rules. In addition, he enjoyed the company of others, enjoyed work, and for a long time had been known as a "helper" in the neighborhood. Each day, finishing his work, he went to the home of "Mr. Jonas," a double amputee, who lived alone in a dark apartment, full of the reminders of a lifetime of collecting. Mr. Jonas had a home health aide who came for 3 hours each day, to help him into the wheelchair, to help him wash, and to prepare some food. However, for Mr. Jonas, the high point of the day was my father's arrival, with news of the community and the synagogue. Most important was the ritual cooking of the split pea soup, which my father prepared for Mr. Jonas every other day. How he loved that soup and the stories about the friends. Mr. Jonas, with no children, had found a solution to continuing to live in the community. This helping model has found adherents in both congregate housing advocates (sharing a house with provision of services) and community sharing plans, where people remain in their own homes but create a "community" where residents provide help for each other when needed.

The solution was not simple for my father. Clearly, he no longer felt safe living alone in his apartment. He was a part of a community, respected, known, and could continue to work in the synagogue. There were not many options. He could find someone who could live with him in the apartment, a "helper," or apply to a long-term care institution, a "nursing home." After some discussion with both of his children, he agreed to go to an interview and be put on the waiting list at a long-term care institution that followed the practices of his tradition. He was acquainted with the Home and had visited friends there. He was fortunate, for the waiting list for men was not long, and within 3 months, he was offered a room.

Moving is always difficult. However, to leave behind all the belongings and memories of a lifetime, now crammed into a small 3-room elderly housing apartment, was extremely hard. There were the books, piled high in the bookcases. The leather-bound collection of the "Papers of the Presidents," purchased when the children were young; religious books and Passover Haggadah's with beautiful pictures; and albums of pictures with memories of the early years in New York with his first wife, on family occasions, with clippings of important events (like the visit to the United States by the King and Queen of England in 1939).

In the kitchen were the old pots, some dented and stained. The meat grinder, which bolted to the edge of the kitchen table, had ground the delicious meat to be stewed with onions and tomatoes. On the shelves was the large seder plate used for so many years and the blue and white china (the few unchipped dishes that were left from the original dishes), wedding gifts to my father and my mother, his first wife. In the corner were the blue glass "movie" dishes, which were collected after so many Sunday films. On the bed in the bedroom were the crocheted spread and the small doilies that his wife had made.

The children did not want or need any of these things, and they could not, of course, be moved to the small room at the Home that would be shared with another person. These rooms were small; closet space was limited to a small wall closet, which many residents supplemented with a portable open closet with hangers. There was a bureau, a small chair, and room for a television or radio. For my father, this was sufficient. Financial issues were not problematic. He had enough funds to enter the Home, and with his social security check, he could receive a small allowance each month. Burial provisions were arranged. It was stipulated on entry that if he were to "spend down" his funds, he would be supported by Medicaid.

My father's general optimism, his love of people and a community, his religious faith, and his desire to work and to help were supplemented by another quality. Since he was a child, he had played the violin "by ear." As an adult, he continued to play, for his and his family's pleasure, for meetings and events at the synagogue, and in his last years, for "old people" in nursing homes. Joined by a friend from the synagogue, he played "quartets," using recordings to supplement the 2 violins. When he left for the nursing home, he composed a song, "While you are alive, live fully. Because life does not go on forever." He added this song to his repertoire of religious and folk songs, very familiar to the population of the nursing home, and became known in the Home for his playing and his participation and singing in the religious ceremony each day. In this way, his desire to work, to be part of a community, and to "help" were all fulfilled in this new setting. Further, he had to admit that cleaning the small apartment, shopping, and cooking had become increasingly more difficult. Now, the setting of the nursing home, with the clean room, the feeling of safety, and what he thought of as the "wonderful meals" were like a dream come true: being taken care of, in a religious setting, and with the possibility of realizing his most important goals.

Each week, in addition to other activities, the Home had a dance program for the residents. Soon my father was attending the dances and was much sought after as a partner by the (mostly single) older women (who form the majority of residents in long-term care institutions). One woman proved especially attractive. "Molly" loved to dance, "to be held," and to take walks, and she enjoyed my father's company. After a 6-month courtship, (which was much discussed by other residents of the Home), my father and Molly decided to marry. It was a grand affair. All of the family attended, and all the residents who could come to the large dining hall with walkers, wheelchairs, and canes, or with assistance from home health aides, were at the ceremony, in the large synagogue. Afterwards, they sang, danced, and ate, joining the family at the celebration. (the event is recorded on a film "Jumping Night in the Garden of Eden" [my father was 91 years old]). In that year, he began to have trouble breathing, and walking became increasingly difficult. In order to receive adequate care, he was moved from the more independent floor to a room, which provided more skilled nursing. It was a wrench for the 2 newlyweds to be separated, but they continued to spend time together in my father's new room. Suffering from congestive heart failure, my father was soon receiving oxygen, and he was provided with a special mattress to avoid bedsores and increasing help in toileting, walking, and so on. His appetite declined, and although the staff was well meaning, the food trays that were delivered at each meal were too full of food that could not be eaten.

Because my father retained his optimism and will to live, the staff decided to wean him off oxygen and generally to encourage more activity. It was difficult for the staff to accept the fact that my father was failing and that his life expectancy was now short, not unusual for a staff that is concerned and feels close to the residents. He died within 6 weeks of his move. It was a great loss to the family and to all those who knew and loved him. For his new wife, it was a special kind of loss. She explained: "While I was married to your father, I was a somebody; everyone admired him and me as well. And now, I am a 'nobody' again."

Everyone has a unique history, personality, needs, and abilities. What was available to my father for long-term care at this time admirably suited his needs, his wishes, and his financial abilities. For him, it was the "golden age."

A PERSONAL ACCOUNT: THE THIRD GENERATION

My husband and I, married 62 years, are retired professionals. We have 4 children, 5 grandchildren, and 3 great grandchildren. Except for 1 son and his family, all live in other parts of the country. All are educated and working, but with small houses, busy lives, and modest incomes, and they do not have the resources to take care of elderly parents. Nor do their parents wish to live with them!

Until our 80s, we were active, fairly healthy, and vigorous. The various ailments of aging then began to appear: arthritis, difficulty with walking, and a general diminution of energy. Friends and family who had moved to continuing care communities urged us to do the same. However, living in a 1-story house (after 40 years in a large 3-storied Victorian) seemed to provide for comfortable and safe living. Home care always seemed an option if there was need for it. We had pensions and some savings and a long-term care policy that provided (after increasing costs) for about one-third of the costs of nursing home or home care (we did not choose to have inflation riders).

Then, the unexpected. (Or should it have been "the expected"?) It is rare to enter one's 80s without the signs of aging. My husband, becoming increasingly more fatigued with ankle swelling, loss of appetite, and general lethargy, was diagnosed with kidney failure. Diagnosis and treatment required a hospital stay and afterward a short stay in a rehabilitation unit. This was very difficult for him (and for his spouse), traveling each day to the various hospitals. Returning home, short-term visiting nurse and physical therapy services covered under Medicare provided some assistance. After a month of driving from home to the kidney dialysis unit 3 afternoons a week, he used "the ride," provided by public transportation for disabled people, except for the days of physician visits.

At this point, the continuing care (or life care) community began to have some appeal.

THE CONTINUING CARE COMMUNITY

The continuing care or life care community is an alternative to home care, assisted living, and nursing home for the middle- and upper-income aged. In existence for over 100 years, these communities were originally church-sponsored groups. Most people who entered these communities were without family and turned over their assets to the institutions, in exchange for a safe and secure caring environment. Since the mid-1900s, these organizations have become mostly for-profit and have grown in number and popularity. The continuum of care provided by the continuing care retirement community (CCRC) encourages the entrance of the resident into independent living, providing a continuum of care within the same familiar community, as the person ages and requires increasing care. There is usually an entrance fee and a monthly fee that is inclusive of some meals, activities, housing, and some of the costs. Some additional costs may be incurred under the insurance plan if the resident uses home care, assisted living, or nursing home care.

What seemed more than adequate, even desirable, to my father when he moved to a long-term care institution was not a consideration for my husband and me, nor most of the people we knew, professionals and business people, active and living in their own homes. We could imagine living in an apartment with pictures on the walls, light and a good view, good meals, activities, a library, and the association with active people of our own age and interests. This included the security of long-term care provided when needed, with the move to assisted living and nursing home if it were necessary. Because the continuing care community focuses on the entry of elders when they are active and well, the resident, knowing that he/she will age, often does not envision the nature of the changes that age will bring. In any case, the "greening" of the nursing home has provided an idea that the rigid medical format of the long-term care institution can be changed by the application of new thinking about the freedom of residents and the way in which care is administered. This is the hope and provides the optimism with which the entry into the continuing care community can be viewed.

The continuing care community is experiencing some of the debits of its own success. With good "wellness" care, and attention to activity, elders in these institutions tend to live long and healthy lives. As people live longer, they also succumb to age changes and require increased assistance. The aged population, 85 years and older, is the fastest growing group (centenarians are not a rarity!). The CCRC finds that it must augment its component of home health aids and other home care features to care for the aged population. This requires increasing supervision with the hiring of outside personnel to meet the needs (as well as increasing costs). In addition, the appearance of canes, walkers, and wheelchairs in the community, where at first there were none, is not conducive to selling the product as independent active living, to a younger generation. Will the baby boomers, as they turn 65 years and older, be interested in living in communities with the elderly residents?

THE YOUNGEST GENERATION

Our oldest daughter is 61 years of age. She is well educated and works as a professional in demanding and interesting work. She has a son and 2 young grandchildren and cannot even imagine a situation in which she would live with her family. She is a part of that baby boomer generation that will greatly increase the ranks of the elderly, those aged 65 years and older. This is a generation that has benefited from economic growth, increased educational access, and an expectation of a surfeit of consumer goods. They jog, do yoga, exercise, and continue to work. Like their children, they wear blue jeans and casual clothes. They have been politically active and vocal. Like many of their parents, they like to think of options available to them. They want to live in a community that provides for active living with educated and accomplished residents and that provides for security and health care. They want a pleasant, bright, and roomy home. Although they could divest themselves of some of their furniture, books, paintings, and other belongings, they would like to continue to have some of their favorite possessions with them.

CONFRONTING THE CHALLENGES

The oldest generation experienced both risks and benefits. If they had children, and the children lived nearby or could assist them, they were satisfied that this was a good solution for the problems accompanying aging. However, if they did not have children, siblings, or other family that could assist them, they were helpless, without funds, and without any security from government or other sources. For some, the religious community provided assistance.

Although my father, as a working man who did not accumulate personal wealth, needed assistance when he was old and alone and did not choose to live with his children, he had the support of social security and a "safety net." The cost of long-term care was affordable under those circumstances. If, like Mr. Jonas, he had chosen to stay at home, home care and the help of friends could have provided assistance.

For the next generation of middle-class professionals, this was not sufficient. We wanted to preserve enough of our way of life, despite difficulties that accompanied aging. Like the next generation, our children, we believed we had a fairly secure retirement. We owned a house and even had some savings. We felt protected until 2008 to 2009 when housing values and investment portfolios shrank and put that security at risk.

In this personal account of 3 generations as they aged, were their experiences only "personal troubles"? Alternatively, were they social problems that required a renewed concern and sense of responsibility for the diverse aged population and its need for care?

FURTHER READINGS

Bennet R, Gurland B, Morris I, et al, editors. Continuing care retirement communities: political social and financial issues. J of Housing for the Elderly 1985;13(1):2.

Gross J. Choosing long term care: advice from an expert. New York Times. September 29, 2008.

Mills CW. The sociological imagination. New York: Oxford University Press; 1959.

Rose A, de Benedictus T, Russell D. Continuing care retirement communities. Available at: www.helpguide.org. 2009. Accessed February 1, 2009.

REFERENCE

1. Myerhoff B. Number our days. New York: Simon and Schuster; 1978. p. 2–5.

Looking Ahead in Long-Term Care: The Next 50 Years

Karen M. Robinson, DNS, PMHCNS-BC, FAAN[a],*,
Susan C. Reinhard, PhD, RN, FAAN[b]

KEYWORDS

• Long-term care • Future • Aging • Trends • Community

One way to think about where the next 50 years will bring us in long-term services and supportive care is to first look back 50 years to gain some perspective. Where were we 50 years ago? The year was 1958, just past the mid-point of the twentieth century:

- Life expectancy was 69.6 years.
- The first Baby Boomers, born in 1946, were 12 years old; this generation will become the "Sandwich Generation," the caregivers of today's older adults.
- There was no Medicare, no Medicaid.
- The nursing home industry was in its infancy, with little, if any, public financing.

American Association of Retired Persons was created by Ethel Percy Andrus, a retired school principal, who at 74 years of age was prompted to act when visiting a retired teacher living in a chicken coop because of having such a meager pension.

Eight years into a new millennium, the world is beginning to recognize that we need to prepare for an aging society. Unless the birth rate rises, our society will continue to age, even if life expectancy does not increase further. At the same time, during the next 50 years, we may see the following:

- Reduced levels of disability among older adults, if the obesity epidemic is reversed.
- Personalized health information, sometimes based on genetic analysis, that helps target lifelong health promotion and disease prevention.
- More livable communities that better support people as they age and need more accessible housing and transportation.
- In-home technology that makes chores easier, and personal care assistance more readily available, perhaps with robotics.

[a] University of Louisville School of Nursing, HSC K Building, Room 4039, Louisville, KY 40292, USA
[b] AARP Public Policy Institute, Center to Champion Nursing in America, 601 E. Street, NW, Washington, DC 20049, USA
* Corresponding author.
E-mail address: kmrobi01@louisville.edu (K.M. Robinson).

We see these trends now, although we cannot predict how they will play out over the next 5 decades. This article reviews how current trends related to chronic illness, care coordination, home- and community-based services, and family caregiving may shape the next 50 years in our long-term care system. Implications for nursing's leadership are highlighted.

CURRENT DEMOGRAPHICS AND COSTS OF CARE

It is well established that Americans are aging. Life expectancy for a child born in 2000 is about 30 years longer than that for a child born a century ago. That is good not bad news. Older adults are a natural resource, maybe our only growing natural resource.

The older population will more than double between 2002 and 2030, from 35.6 million to 71.5 million, and almost 1 in 5 people will be 65 years or older.[1] On reaching age 65 years, the average person in America today can expect to live an additional 18 years or 6 years longer than people aged 65 years lived in 1940.[2] Declining fertility rates, longer life expectancy, and aging of the baby boomers are among many factors that contribute to the aging of America's population. The oldest of 79 million baby boomers, born between 1946 and 1964, will reach age 65 years in just 2 years. The long-term care system will not feel the effect of aging baby boomers as quickly as the Medicare and Social Security program. That is because older people typically do not need long-term care until they are well into their 70s and 80s.[3]

The imminent retirement of the baby boom generation has spurred researchers, policymakers, and advocates to think anew about America's health care system, especially about its cost. The cost of health care is staggering. In 1970, America spent $73 billion on health care, including government, insurers, employers, and individuals. By 2003, the figure was $1.6 trillion.[4] Health care costs for American families continue to consume an increasing share of income and economic resources.

According to the Congressional Budget Office, the widespread use of new medical services and technologies is the most important factor driving long-term spending growth—across all ages. In fact, surprisingly, the aging of the population accounts for a very small portion of this growth well past the next 50 years (see **Fig. 1**).

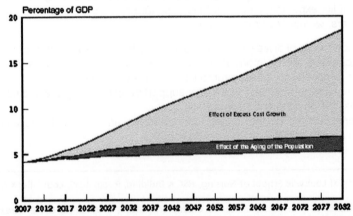

Fig. 1. Sources of growth in projected federal spending on Medicare and Medicaid Congressional Budget Office, The Outlook for Spending on Health Care and Long-Term Care Presentation to the National Governors Association's Health and Human Service's Committee, February 2008. (*Data from* Congressional Budget Office. The long-term outlook for health care spending. Available at: http://www.cbo.gov/ftpdocs/87xx/doc8758/MainText.3.1.shtml. Accessed April 21, 2009.)

Costs in our national system of health care have been difficult to contain. In the next 50 years, the primary challenge for the US health care system is to transform it to ensure access to more affordable, higher-quality care, including long-term care. Long-term care, known as "long-term services and supports," needs to be more inclusive of all settings of care, yet currently it is not covered by Medicare nor most private health insurance plans. The cost of these services can be the single greatest threat to the health and financial security of older people; about 16% of people who turned 65 years in 2005 needed at least $100,000 to manage the costs of their long-term care.[5]

CHRONIC ILLNESS: WILL WE MANAGE IT BETTER?

Medicare will pay for acute exacerbations of chronic illness, not the full range of care for chronic illness and not long-term care that involves more personal care of persons who need help with activities of daily living (ADLs) (bathing, dressing, toileting, transferring, and eating). However, understanding the population served by Medicare in the next 50 years can be helpful in thinking about how future older adults may differ from those we serve now. Current trends project a profile of our future Medicare population.[6]

First, we expect to see an increase in the treated prevalence of chronic illness. Increased treatments will result from the increase in obesity among Americans as well as advances in the diagnosis and treatment of illnesses and new definitions of diseases. Over the past 15 years, the number of people in the United States with diagnosed diabetes has more than doubled, reaching 14.6 million in 2005, while another 6.2 million probably have the disease without knowing it. During the past 30 years, the prevalence of obesity among US adults has approximately doubled. In 2005 to 2006, more than 34% of adults aged 20 years or older were obese and at increased risk for heart disease, high blood pressure, diabetes, and other illnesses.[6]

Second, we will see a more diverse Medicare population. Today, the older than-65 years population is about 6% Hispanic and 3% Asian. However, the cohort that will age into Medicare beginning in 2020 is 9% Hispanic and 4% Asian.[6]

Finally, aging boomers' higher levels of educational attainment are likely to spur them to take a more active role in health care decision making. Boomers also have fewer children, and those children are more likely to be geographically dispersed from their parents, perhaps decreasing their ability to undertake caregiving tasks. The Institute of Medicine[7] speculates that, given their high rate of health provider visits, the baby boomers may have greater expectations about care or may be more aggressive about treating their illnesses than previous generations of older adults.

These differences will affect the health care system as consumers become more active in their own care. Increased diversity in the population will become more important, with language barriers posing some problems and some health characteristics driving particular concerns. For example, the growing population of Hispanics has higher diabetes prevalence, more ADL limitations, and less insurance coverage than those of other populations.[6] These differences should stimulate corresponding changes in the health and long-term care systems.

The Institute of Medicine[7] noted in its recent report, *Retooling for an Aging America*, that the health care needs of an aging population are different. For instance, among the population as a whole, there were 329 physician office visits per 100 persons; but for those aged between 65 and 74 years, the frequency nearly doubled to 647 and increased even further in the 75-and-over population to 768. Days of hospital care per 100 persons were 55.4 for the entire population but 140 for 65- to 74-year-olds and 259 for those aged 75 years and older.[7] These differences translate into projected use increases. This increased use of health care will provide increased demand for nurses and other health care providers and an urgent need for consumers to self-manage their care.

Active Consumers

One of the salient features of chronic disease is that consumers and their family care-givers can take many active steps to manage their own care. For example, diet and exercise can help a person with diabetes avoid acute manifestations of the disease, or taking blood pressure medications regularly can keep hypertension under control. Recognizing and acting on warning signs and symptoms can avoid the need for emergency care later. Absence of alcohol and cigarette abuse before age 50 years was found to be the most important protective factors for successful aging.[8] Not all consumers will be able to understand or will take control of their own health. An important component of chronic disease management will be an appreciation of the need to engage, activate, and educate consumers about their illness and build the competence and confidence for consumers to take charge of their own health.

Better Tools to Manage Chronic Disease

In the future, people with chronic illness will have access to information to manage their disease. Good communication between providers and consumers is just now beginning but will become critical. Some chronic care management programs organize group meetings among people with the same chronic disease to share information, provide motivation, and support in maintaining healthy behaviors. Providing consumers and their caregivers with access to information about resources in the community will help maintain function and independence.

Technology

Using the Internet can be helpful in managing chronic illness; trends suggest this competency will continue to be important. Computer and Internet use among the older population is on the increase. Initiatives have been developed to erase the "gray" digital divide whereby many older people miss out on the benefits that computers and the Internet can provide.

Reasons why older people do not use computers and the Internet have received practical solutions, highlighting the importance of changing misconceptions about computers, providing better information about what computers are, what they can do, and how they can be of real practical use.[9] In a field test of household Internet usage, 89% of 93 families needed support from the computer help desk in the first year they used the Internet. The most technically involved member of the family was called upon to become a mentor to assist other family members with technical support. Often the family member with the most skill was a teenager and became the person in the family others turned to for technology. The teenager benefited from this role, influenced the household's acceptance of technology, and represented an important link between households and use of latest technology. The role is also an example of strengths observed in the use of intergenerational relationships.[10]

Dramatic examples of household helpers will occur as Japan builds a new generation of robot companions. These robots are designed to serve as assistants around the house. Current designs identify up to 8 family members by face or voice, remind you when to take your medicine, make an appointment, and will send photographs of an intruder to your mobile phone if someone breaks into your house. Japan and American firms have their eye on the same market: robots for home health care.

As baby boomers hit retirement age, the need to monitor and assist seniors will create increased demand.[11]

Japan, which has long been fascinated with the robot, is making machines that look and act like human beings with the technology of artificial intelligence. US firms, however, are instead emphasizing products targeted to specific service tasks, like mowing lawns, cleaning pools, and taking vital signs. Since 2001, Japan has spent $210 million on research to deploy robots to support its aging workforce. Goals set forth are that robots should be able to straighten a room by the end of 2008, make beds by 2013, and help with baths and meals by 2025. In the next 50 years, robots could be the biggest technological revolution since personal computers and the Internet.[11]

Care Coordination

As care needs become ever more complex in the future, well-prepared geriatric professionals will be increasingly in demand to coordinate that care. Care coordination has been defined as "the deliberate integration of patient care activities between 2 or more participants involved in a patient's care to facilitate the appropriate delivery of health care services."[12] Care coordination links people with special health care needs and their families to services and resources in a coordinated effort to maximize the potential of the client and provide optimal health care.[12,13] Care coordination is complicated, because there is no single point of entry to multiple systems of care, and complex criteria determine the availability of funding and services among public and private payers. Sociocultural and economic barriers to coordination of care exist and negatively affect families and care professionals.[14] Nurse care coordinators have a vital role in the process of care coordination. Nurses are recognized as leaders in providing care coordination[15] and have great interest in supporting better methods for providing care coordination to persons with multiple chronic conditions.

Driven by the need to increase value to the consumers and payers of health care, care coordination services will be provided by the most cost-effective clinician. Integrating baccalaureate and masters-prepared nurses into interdisciplinary treatment teams as part of disease management programs is a way to reduce costs of health care.[16] Over the past decade, many health plans have instituted or expanded disease management programs for enrollees with chronic conditions and case management programs for the more seriously ill. Most of these programs have identified the nurse as the logical team leader and provider of coordinated care. In disease management programs, nurses as members of the interdisciplinary team have taken leadership to help patients self-manage their own illnesses.

Interdisciplinary Care

As care needs of older adults become more complex, alternative care delivery systems need to be developed. The vision of care in the future is that services need to be delivered more efficiently.[7] A common feature identified in new models of care indicates that care delivered by an interdisciplinary team holds the most promise for improving quality and outcomes.

Interdisciplinary team care occurs when providers from different disciplines collaboratively manage the care of the patient. Providers may include primary care physicians, registered nurses, social workers, physical therapists, pharmacists, occupational therapists, recreational therapists, dieticians, home care providers, personal care attendants, and drivers. Team members communicate regularly with each other about their patients.[7] This interdisciplinary approach is believed to help support quality care by improving communication among providers and their patients.

New models promote care that is seamless across various care delivery sites, and, therefore, all providers need to have access to patients' health information when needed. Technology such as electronic health records and remote monitoring will be used to support interdisciplinary patient care and care coordination.[7] In the "person-centered care" framework, older persons need to be active partners in their own care, unless they are too frail, mentally or physically, to participate. The interdisciplinary team includes partnership with the patient and family, whereby the team's purpose is to increase participation by the patient and family in decision making. By including the patient and family in decision making, patients can improve their health, reduce unnecessary treatments, and reduce the need for reliance on both formal and informal caregivers.

What barriers have existed to prevent formation of interdisciplinary teams in modern health care? Currently, care is delivered by multiple providers who are often not linked in any way. The first barrier preventing team formation has to do with time: time for the providers to get together to discuss patient care and time for the family to meet with the provider. The fast-paced, multispecialist approach in our modern care system has triggered a crisis in care. A second barrier is communication.[17] The real challenge is to achieve clear, open communication when providers are all extremely busy. Communication is critical when gathering data and successfully implementing a treatment plan. Communication needs to be coordinated by 1 person so that many different clinicians do not have to ask the patient the same questions repeatedly. There has been a diffusion of responsibility with no one person identified who will coordinate care. Communication remains one of the most important influences on the quality of care and can determine the nature of clinical outcomes.[18]

The current health care workforce lacks key competencies necessary for work in interdisciplinary teams. Over the coming 50 years, the nature of health care will change dramatically. New multidisciplinary relationships will develop to include new consumer and clinician relationships to provide patient-centered care.[19] Another needed competency will be to use quality improvement skills to reduce errors. Education for the health professions is in need of drastic change; rather than occurring in individual silos, interdisciplinary experiences must be used in clinical education. Health care clinicians will need to develop competencies to lead interdisciplinary teams and strive to implement evidence-based practice to improve the quality of health care.[20] Providers will need to be trained to work in interdisciplinary teams, and financing and delivery systems need to support this interdisciplinary approach.

The health care workforce will have a central role in treating chronic illness and will be at the front line of efforts to change this trend of fragmented, acute care to focus on public health initiatives that make our population healthier. Chronic illness care along the continuum demands greater cooperation between physicians and nurses. The nurse's role varies from being a teammate to being a full partner in the care of seriously ill patients. Studies conducted by Ohman-Strickland and colleagues[21] indicate that practices employing nurse practitioners perform as well if not better than practices employing physicians only and those employing physician assistants. Thus, stakeholders must be open to multiple and diverse options for successful models of care. The historical practice of training health professions in silos is inappropriate for a delivery system that emphasizes chronic care.

LONG-TERM CARE: HOME- AND COMMUNITY-BASED CARE

Considerable evidence suggests that the prevalence of disability and need for long-term care may be significantly decreased in the next 50 years. Several factors lend optimism for health trends that may lower the future cost of nursing homes and other expenditures.[22] The over-riding trend is the move toward home- and community-based care, including the design of communities to support aging in communities and better support of family caregivers.

Over the next 50 years, a paradigm shift will occur in how we think about long-term care facilities. Older people want the same chance that younger people have, to choose autonomy in their own care control, individuality, and continuity in a meaningful personal life. These values are held with higher regard than is safety. Older people want to live in a home-like setting that allows their own decision making such as they have made for themselves over their lifetime—when to get up, eat breakfast, take a bath, and go to bed. Autonomy will be given, such as being able to choose activities of great interest—reading a book, listening to music, taking a walk, dancing, and telling stories. People will continue to prefer to get care where they live, rather than to live in an institution that focuses on care. They will desire to have personal items collected over a lifetime as part of their surroundings and to have a regular, consistent caregiver who knows and understands these preferences.

This paradigm shift will transform the long-term care system from an acute-care, medical model system managed by physicians and nurses to a consumer-directed model. This culture change must de-emphasize the institution and give rise to person-centered care. Long-term care facilities must become more homelike, operated under the imperative to honor residents' desires, and allow flexibility in sleeping and eating schedules, preferences in bathing, and choices of activities. Facilities must focus on quality of life and offer dignity and autonomy along with quality care.[23]

Livable Communities

To live at home, we will need more livable communities. We are already moving in that direction. States and local governments have taken the initiative for all builders to include at least 3 features in new houses to build accessible communities. These trends are related to 3 changes: no steps at the entrance, a bathroom on the ground floor, and wider doorways. Some states' building codes offer builders incentives to provide 36-in-wide doors and hallways, a bathroom on the first floor, an entry with no steps, light switches, outlets at wheelchair level, and reinforced walls in the bathroom to support a grab bar.

These features allow people to live independently in their own homes for as long as possible. Fulfilling these requirements can add $200 to $1,000 to the cost of building a home, but it is cheaper to build it correctly the first time rather than retrofitting it later. Over the next 50 years, these design features will become standard nationwide. Housing trends such as these allow seniors to live independently rather than having to move into an assisted-living facility or nursing home. It reduces the personal and social costs of having to relocate to institutional living.[24]

Family Caregivers

Family-based caregiving assistance is the primary source of long-term care for older persons with chronic illness. Unpaid caregivers provide the majority of services and supports received by persons with chronic illness of all ages. In November 2006, between 30 million and 38 million adult caregivers (age 18 years and older) provided care to adults with at least 1 limitation in an ADL. Caregivers provided an average of 21 hours of care per week or 1,080 h/y at an average value of $9.63/h. The value of this unpaid care is estimated at $350 billion/y in 2006.[25]

The contributions of caregivers are not only the foundation of the long-term care system but are also an important component of the US economy. Frequent help with basic personal care reduces the likelihood of nursing home use among persons aged 70 years and older over a 2-year period by about 60%.[26] Without family help, both state and federal long-term care budgets would be overwhelmed by the need for services, because the nation does not have a sufficient supply of direct care workers to replace informal caregivers.[27] Caregiver stress is a strong predictor of nursing home entry. Reducing key stresses (such as physical strain and financial hardship) on caregivers will reduce nursing home admission.[28] Over the next 50 years, it will be essential to prevent family caregivers from becoming overwhelmed by the demands placed on them.

Trends of increased longevity in our population will mean changes in family structures and relationships. The family systems perspective means that changes such as aging that affect one member also affect the whole family. Longer life spans mean that 4- and 5-generation extended families will be more common. Aging couples will have 30 to 40 years ahead together after their children leave home. As the population ages, the likelihood of living alone will increase, more for women than for men because women live longer. Over the past years, the percentage of 65+ population living in a nursing home has remained relatively constant and small (less than 5%), but the percentage increases dramatically with age to 18.2% for persons 85+.[1] The young old at retirement will be involved in caregiving for their old-old parents.[29]

Forward-looking trends and practices in family caregiver support will be implemented to bolster caregiving families and improve the quality of care for adults who receive long-term care at home. Three accepted trends with important implications to address the needs of family caregivers are as follows: caregiver assessment, consumer direction in family caregiver support services, and collaborations between the aging network and health care system.[30]

Caregiver Assessment

One key to improving outcomes in community settings is not just assessing the older person with chronic illness but the family caregiver as well. Systematic assessment of family caregiver needs has been implemented because of recognition of the fundamental need to sustain caregiving families and keep them healthy. Use of a single, universal assessment tool for long-term care clients, including family caregivers, will be implemented in most states. Caregiver assessments are used to tailor care plans and support services to meet the needs of family caregivers. Future programs for long-term services and support will mandate a caregiver assessment.

Consumer Direction

Consumer-directed service options will be the predominant model of long-term services and supports. Family members, neighbors, and friends will be paid either for direct services or for coordinating services. Consumer-directed options for caregivers now include respite care (such as in-home care, adult day care, or weekend or overnight stays in a long-term care facility) as well as supplemental services (such as home modifications, yard work, chore services, and assistive devices). All states will provide both options, which include a list of approved providers and goods from which caregivers may choose or allow caregivers to hire someone privately.

COLLABORATIONS ON CAREGIVING BETWEEN THE AGING NETWORK AND THE HEALTH CARE SYSTEM

Partnerships will be common between the Area Agencies on Aging and health care providers. Family caregiver support programs will reach caregivers before they experience adverse effects by proactively identifying them in primary care physician offices, rather than waiting for caregivers to seek help or provide care alone. Thus, this support keeps caregivers healthy and delays institutionalization for those receiving care for as long as possible. These 3 trends will be implemented, because they adopt a more family-centered perspective in assessing needs and delivering services.

SUMMARY

In the next 50 years, nurses need to demonstrate leadership in moving the country forward to ensure that all of us will have more effective chronic care and more humane long-term care. We can create what we ourselves would prefer—not fragmented care, burdened families, and institutionalization. We can promote programs and policies that put people and their families in the center, with nurses and other health professionals supporting them in homes and communities. The time to start is now.

REFERENCES

1. Centers for Disease Control and Prevention. Public health and aging: Trends in aging: United States and worldwide. 2003. Available at: http://www.cdc.gov/mmwr/preview/mmwrhtml/mm5206a2.htm. Accessed September 12, 2007.
2. Centers for Disease Control and Prevention. Fast stats A to Z. Available at: http://www.cdc.gov/nchs/fastats/deaths.htm. Accessed September 27, 2007.
3. Stevenson DG. Planning for the future–long term care and the 2008 election. N Engl J Med 2008;358(19):1985–7.
4. Smith C, Cowan C, Sensenig A, et al. Health spending growth slows in 2003. Health Aff 2005;24(1):185–94.
5. Kemper P, Komisar HL, Alecxih L. Long term care over an uncertain future: what can retirees expect? Inquiry 2005;335–50.
6. Medicare Payment Advisory Commission. Increasing the value of Medicare: report to the Congress on medicare payment policy. Washington, DC: MEDPAC; 2008.
7. Institute of Medicine. Retooling for an aging America: building the health care workforce. Washington, DC: National Academies Press; 2008.
8. Vaillant GE, Mukamal K. Successful aging. Am J Psychiatry 2001;158(6):839–47.
9. Morris AJ, Goodman, Brading H. Internet use and non-use: views of older users. Universal Access in the Information Society 2007;6(1):43–57.
10. Kiesler S, Zdaniuk B, Lundmark V, et al. Troubles with the Internet: the dynamics of help at home. Int J Hum Comp 2000;15(4):323–51.
11. Baker K. Why should we be friends? As Japan builds a new generation of robot companions, US firms focus on pragmatics. Newsweek. August 18–25, 2008.
12. McDonald K, Sundaram V, Bravata DM, et al. Closing the quality gap: a critical analysis of quality improvement strategies. In: Care coordination. Rockville (MD): Agency for Healthcare Research and Quality; 2007.
13. Committee on children with disabilities. Care coordination: integrating health and related systems of care for children with special health care needs. Pediatrics 1999;104(4):978–81.
14. Kodner D, Kyriacou C. Fully integrated care for frail elderly: two American models. Int J Integr Care 2000;1:e08. (Available at: http://www.pubmedcentral.nih.gov/articlerender.fcgi?artid=1533997).
15. Bodenheimer T, MacGregor K, Stothart N. Nurses as leaders in chronic care. Br Med J 2005;330(7492):612–3.

16. Disease Management Association of America (DMAA). DMAA literature database. Available at: http://www.dmaa.org/dmlibrary/web%20Edition-%20 April%202004.doc. Accessed March 7, 2008.
17. Penson RT, Kyriakou H, Zuckerman D, et al. Teams: communication in multidisciplinary care. Oncologist 2006;11(5):520–6.
18. Boyle D, Miller P, Forbes-Thompson S. Communication and end of life care in the intensive care unit: patient, family, and clinician outcomes. Crit Care Nurs Q 2005; 28:302–16.
19. Sievers B, Wolf S. Teams: communication in multidisciplinary care. Clin Nurse Spec 2006;20(2):75–80.
20. Benedict L, Robinson K, Holder C. Clinical nurse specialist practice within the acute care for elders interdisciplinary team model. Clin Nurse Spec 2006;20(5): 248–51.
21. Ohman-Strickland PA, Orzano AJ, Hudson SV, et al. Quality of diabetes care in family medicine practices: influence of nurse-practitioners and physician's assistants. Ann Fam Med 2008;6(1):14–22. Available at: http://www.annfammed.org/ cgi/content/abstract/6/1/14.
22. Burton H, Singer, Manton K. The effects of health changes on projections of health service needs for the elderly population of the United States. Proc Natl Acad Sci U S A 1998;95(26):15618–22.
23. Alliance for Health Reform. Changing the nursing home culture 2008. Washington, DC.
24. AARP. Reimagining America: How America can grow old and prosper. In: AARP's Blueprint for the future, Washington, DC: AARP; 2005.
25. Gibson MJ, Houser A. Valuing the invaluable: a new look at the economic value of family caregiving. Issue Brief. Washington, DC: AARP; 2007. p. IB–82.
26. Lo Sasso A, Johnson R. Does informal care from adult children reduce nursing home admissions for the elderly? Inquiry 2002;39:279–97.
27. National Commission for Quality Long Term Care. The long term care workforce: can the crisis be fixed? Washington, DC: Institute for the Future of Aging Services; 2007.
28. Spillman B, Long SK. Does high caregiver stress lead to nursing home entry?. Washington, DC: United States Department of Health and Human Services; 2007.
29. Gavan, CS. Successful aging families: a challenge for nurses. Holist Nurs Pract; 17(1):11–18.
30. Fox-Grage W, Gibson MJ. Ahead of the curve: emerging trends and practice in family caregiver support. In Brief. Washington, DC: AARP; 2006.

Index

Note: Page numbers of article titles are in **boldface** type.

A

Access, to healthcare, hospice, 236–238
    as a controversial issue, 236
    barriers and enablers of, 236–237
    policy barriers to, 237–238
African Americans, disparities in long-term healthcare, **179–185**
Aging, future outlook on long-term care, **253–262**
    chronic illness, better management of, 255–258
    collaborations on caregiving, 260–261
    current demographics and costs of care, 254–255
    home and community-based, 258–260
Aging in place, technology systems to enhance home care, **239–246**
    e-learning, 244–245
    electronic documentation system, 241–242
    telemedicine, 242–243
    telephony, 243–244
Alzheimer's disease, caregiver burden, three views on, **209–221**
Assessment, by nurse practitioner of pain in nursing home residents, 201–204
Assisted living, disparities in long-term care, **179–185**
    background, 179–180
    chronic disease management, 180–181
    end-of-life issues, 181

B

Bringing the Best to Nursing program, diversity leadership in, 173
Burden, being one at end of life, 225
    caregiver, three views of, **209–221**

C

Caregivers, burden of Alzheimer's disease on, three views of, **209–221**
    questions to ask patients near end of life, 226
    See also Family caregivers.
Certified nursing assistants (CNAs), in nursing homes, diversity and, 171–172
    community partnerships, 174–175
    improving CNA retention, 175–177
Chronic disease, disparities in management of, 180–181
    future outlook for management of, 255–258
        active consumers, 256
        better tools for, 256

Nurs Clin N Am 44 (2009) 263–269
doi:10.1016/S0029-6465(09)00021-8
0029-6465/09/$ – see front matter © 2009 Elsevier Inc. All rights reserved.

nursing.theclinics.com

Moving?

Make sure your subscription moves with you!

To notify us of your new address, find your **Clinics Account Number** (located on your mailing label above your name), and contact customer service at:

E-mail: elspcs@elsevier.com

800-654-2452 (subscribers in the U.S. & Canada)
314-453-7041 (subscribers outside of the U.S. & Canada)

Fax number: 314-523-5170

Elsevier Periodicals Customer Service
11830 Westline Industrial Drive
St. Louis, MO 63146

*To ensure uninterrupted delivery of your subscription, please notify us at least 4 weeks in advance of move.

Printed and bound by CPI Group (UK) Ltd, Croydon, CR0 4YY
08/06/2025
01896873-0007